# BUT NOW I SEE

A MEDICAL INTUITIVE SURGEON'S GUIDE
TO THE MEANING OF YOUR ILLNESS
AND THE SECRETS TO HEALING
CHRONIC AND INCURABLE DISEASE

VERONICA ANDERSON, M.D.

© 2018 by Veronica Anderson

All rights reserved. No part of this book may be reproduced or transmitted in any form or by any means, electronic or mechanical, including photocopying, recording, or by any information storage and retrieval system, except in the case of brief quotations embodied in critical articles and reviews, without prior written permission of the publisher.

Although the author and publisher have made every effort to ensure the accuracy and completeness of information contained in this book, we assume no responsibility for errors, inaccuracies, omissions, or any inconsistency herein.

Printed in the United States of America

Library of Congress Control Number: 2018932628

ISBN Paperback: 978-1-947368-94-1
ISBN eBook: 978-1-947368-60-6

Cover Design: C7 creativezone
Interior Design: Ghislain Viau

BUT
NOW
I
SEE

# Contents

A Letter of Introduction . . . . . . . . . . . . . . . . . . . . . . . vii

Welcome! I was worried you wouldn't show . . . . . . . . . ix

## PART ONE: FORGET THE SCIENCE . . . . . . . . . . . . . . . . . . . 1

**Chapter 1:** Does Your Religion Make You Sick? . . . . . . . 3
    Catholic to Clairvoyant . . . . . . . . . . . . . . . . . . . . . 7

**Chapter 2:** Does Your Doctor Make You Sick? . . . . . . . 13
    Intuition to Industrial: The Problem
      with Modern Medicine . . . . . . . . . . . . . . . . . . 16
    Medical Intuitive: Diagnosing the Spiritual . . . . . . 18

**Chapter 3:** Miracles (Bending the Rules) . . . . . . . . . . . 29

## PART TWO: GET WITH THE YOU-YOU . . . . . . . . . . . . . . . . 37

**Chapter 4:** Your Spirit . . . . . . . . . . . . . . . . . . . . . . . . . 39
    Spiritual Evaluation: Asking Deeper Questions . . . 41
    Build Your Self-Evaluation Skills . . . . . . . . . . . . . 43

**Chapter 5:** Your Mind . . . . . . . . . . . . . . . . . . . . . . . . . 53
    Eight Easy Ways to Stay Sane . . . . . . . . . . . . . . 54

**Chapter 6:** Your Body (Part I) . . . . . . . . . . . . . . . . . . . 71
    Exercise . . . . . . . . . . . . . . . . . . . . . . . . . . . . . . . . . 74
    Diet: What You Eat Is Eating You . . . . . . . . . . . . 82

**Chapter 7:** Your Body (Part II) . . . . . . . . . . . . . . . . . . . 93
    Signaling to the Universe . . . . . . . . . . . . . . . . . . . 93
    Chemical Signals . . . . . . . . . . . . . . . . . . . . . . . . . 97
    Killer Stress . . . . . . . . . . . . . . . . . . . . . . . . . . . . . 101

**REFLECTIONS** . . . . . . . . . . . . . . . . . . . . . . . . . . . . . . . 109

# A Letter of Introduction

Dearly beloved health-seekers,

I know you are here because you are interested in bringing about a transformation in your spiritual, physical, or emotional health. Because I care for your complete health, I am offering you, my reader, a range of FREE and discounted services. By using the unique links within this book, you will receive gifts and discounts worth over $1,000!

My first gift is a meditation (valued at $497) that you can both hear and see: Meditation on Flowers at drveronica.com/flowers/

Also included in this book are FREE health and toxic-exposure assessments:

- Are You Toxic?: drveronica.wufoo.com/forms/are-you-toxic/

- How Healthy Are You?: drveronica.wufoo.com/forms/how-healthy-are-you/

For those who feel they would benefit from more guidance after reading this book, you will find that all these unique links offer samples of my services for half price:
- Living Matrix Health Assessment: drveronica.wufoo.com/forms/special-offer-living-matrix-evaluation-297/
- Full Medical Intuitive Reading: drveronica.wufoo.com/forms/special-offer-full-medical-intuitive-reading/
- Single-Question Reading: drveronica.wufoo.com/forms/special-offer-single-question-reading/
- Health-Creation Meditation: drveronica.wufoo.com/forms/special-offer-health-creation-meditation/

And finally, you can get a $50 discount at the genetic-testing site 23andme.com by visiting 23andme.com/drveronica.

With gratitude, love, and joy,

Dr. Veronica
http://drveronica.com/start-here/

# Welcome! I was worried you wouldn't show...

You *could* have chosen any number of titles from the shelf in the health section and taken the well-trodden path of conventional medicine. Or you could have bypassed books completely and gone to the University of Google or Doctor YouTube. You could also have turned on the TV to watch *The Dr. Oz Show* for little nuggets of health advice that you can share at cocktail parties.

You *could* have chosen to continue to keep focused on what is wrong with your body, its aches, its pains, and its strains. This is something we're all conditioned to do. We are all obsessed with our bodies because pharmaceutical ads and medical advice are everywhere we look.

## But Now I See

But you didn't opt for the usual; instead, you have arrived here, with me. My name is Dr. Veronica Anderson, and I'm so glad you choose this book.

What I want to show you in this book is that your body is only one-third of the wellness pie. Our mind and our spirit make up the whole, but Western medicine—which is too concerned with flesh and bone—often refuses to engage with the mind and spirit, which are dismissed as belonging to the realm of "woo-woo" alternative treatments. This is despite the fact it is clear that conventional medicine doesn't have all the answers. In fact, according to the Centers for Disease Control and Prevention, **one in twenty-five people in the hospital at any given moment, are being treated for hospital-acquired infections.** (Source: cdc.gov/hai/surveillance/index.) This suggests that conventional medicine is making our bodies sicker!

I was a practicing eye surgeon, medically trained in the conventional way; my calling is to help people see. But I am also here, in this life, to help people see in a more figurative sense, and so this book is intended to open your eyes to the importance of your mind and spirit to your bodily health.

We are taught by the "wisdom" of Western medicine to focus on our physical ills. But I believe that a lot of people—way back in their mind somewhere—understand that stress has been causing their problems and making them sick. However,

## Welcome! I was worried you wouldn't show . . .

they've never made it clear how stress does this. I also believe that the fact people in our society have become separated from their emotional and spiritual selves is why illnesses and injuries can linger on, and on, and on.

This book will show you that in order to really heal yourself—which is different from finding a cure—you have to do some emotional and spiritual work. You can get a pill to cure your ailment, but to truly *heal* and move forward, there must be an emotional and a spiritual shift.

**However, if you want me to open your eyes to the possibilities, you must read with an open mind.**

This book contains some ideas that many would consider "out there," and you might be shocked to discover how you are unknowingly contributing to your own illnesses. But I don't set out to offend. Rather, my aim is only to show you new ways of thinking about yourself—your whole self.

You have nothing to lose and everything to gain by being open to possibilities, and I promise we'll have some fun along the way. I want this book to be fun because fun is a health-promoting activity!

What I would like you to gain from reading this book is hope and power. This is a book of true empowerment because it's going to pave the way for you to understand more about yourself—not the *science* of you, but the *spirit* and the *emotions* of you, which are so rarely taken into account by conventional medicine.

I want you to find hope that there are healthcare practitioners out there, like me, who care for hearts and souls, and who can help you. Hope is necessary for a miracle to happen. I'm not talking about the water-into-wine kind of miracle, but the miracles that occur in the self when people shift their thinking and open themselves to something that yesterday seemed impossible. At the end of each chapter, I offer you a gift that will help you discover and enjoy your soul journey, and I hope that by the end of the book you will have gained the miracle of that open mind and the hope and power to be fully well in body, mind, and spirit.

## Part One
# Forget the Science

*"One man's woo-woo, of course,
is another's deeply held belief system."*
—Julia Moskin, US Journalist

"That's just woo-woo!"

When have you heard that? Most likely, you've heard it said about something mystical, something unproven by science. But I'll bet you've probably never heard it said about one of the major religions, even though there's no scientific basis for any of them. Faith is not founded in science; it's founded in knowing in your heart something is true.

Just because we can't prove it, should we just ignore it? I don't think so. Whenever there is a lack of evidence, it may simply mean we're not yet smart enough to figure out how to prove it. Think about it. Woo-woo exists in regular science too. Physicists know dark matter exists because they can see its effects all over the universe; they just have not been able to identify it . . . yet. One day, their tools and understanding may have advanced enough to show us exactly what dark matter is and how it works.

And how much do neurologists know about the brain? Not a whole bunch. With so much more exploration of our brains left to do, how can anyone say for sure that our brains are *not* capable of mind reading or clairvoyance or other psychic phenomena that are often dismissed by the closed-minded as being woo-woo?

Faith in anything ends up being woo-woo, because somebody had to have faith in whatever it was to even go out and study it in the first place. Woo-woo is simply faith in whatever people think is going on in the universe, or our bodies, that they cannot see clearly yet.

Hopefully, then, you're willing to venture with me into the next few chapters to explore a few concepts that may be unrelated to science, but they are critical to your health and wellbeing. There are a bunch of health-science books out there—and more come out every day—yet people are getting sicker, so there must be something missing, right?

So let's get on with it!

# Chapter 1

# Does Your Religion Make You Sick?

Neither of my parents was born Catholic. My mother grew up a Baptist, and my father was raised an African Methodist Episcopal Zionist—both Protestant religions. Then, for I don't know what reason, they decided they were going to follow Catholicism together and raise their children in the Catholic Church.

When my sister was born, two years before I was, they named her Pamela Ophelia. They chose "Pamela" because they liked it, and "Ophelia" because it is the name of my mother's adoptive mother. When it was time for Pamela to be baptized as an infant, the priest gave my parents a hard time because my sister did not have a name in the Catholic

Bible (I say "Catholic Bible," because it has seven more books than the Protestant version). The church didn't want my sister baptized there, so my mother said, "OK then, her name's 'Mary.'" The church didn't seem concerned about the soul of my sister; they were more concerned about following some rule that nobody understood. (I still don't get it, by the way. The Bible is supposed to be the word of God, but somehow the Catholic Bible is different then the other Bibles? People fight wars over this stuff!)

Two years later, I was born and my parents selected the name "Veronica," partly because they liked it, but also because there's a Saint Veronica in the Catholic Bible. Saint Veronica, so the story goes, laid a veil on the face of Jesus, and when she took the veil away, there was a miraculous imprint of his face on the fabric. I'll come back to Veronica and her veil later in this chapter.

So I grew up Catholic and I went to church. But when I was about nine years old, my mother decided to leave the Catholic Church, and so both my sister and I left too.

Many years later, when I got married, I returned to church, but this time it was a traditional African-American–based Baptist church. After Sunday services, the church held a lunch for the congregation, which would have been great had the food options not been incredibly unhealthy. I'm talking, fried chicken, syrupy peach cobbler, and overcooked and heavily salted vegetables. The only salad was made with iceberg lettuce. There was nothing of any nutritional value! It was all so unhealthy that I wondered if the church was trying to send me to Heaven earlier than I wanted to go! But it took me a little longer to realize that what they were feeding my mind was far worse. It felt as if they wanted me to hate myself. They repeatedly said bad things about me and wanted me to believe bad stuff about myself. They wanted to cripple my mind with fear and anger and sadness so that I would need to depend on them.

I was intelligent and curious so when I heard all this trash talk in church, I found it frustrating. I would say, "God created me like this! Why would God create me with a curious nature but think his creation was a bad person?" But whenever I asked questions, people would reply, "Because it says so in the Bible!" Asking deeper questions was not encouraged at all, and I began to wonder if there was more beyond the limited belief system I encountered at church.

As I grew up, I also struggled with the concept of the devil as the red guy with horns and a pitchfork that the church depicted in order to instill fear, especially in children. Do you really think that all powerful, all-loving Creator sat around making a devil just to scare us? Could the Creator really be that mean and small-minded? I believe that the devil was created to oppress—not by God, but by people who wanted to control others. There is evil in the world, but only in people who do a good job at acting like the devil. Believing in "Hell" and "Satan" puts guilt and shame on you, which boils down to the emotion of fear. The Abrahamic religions would have you believe that this is the one and only earthly life you'll have; this life is it. But fear creates stress, and stress kills.

If you don't like what I'm saying, close this book and continue to live in fear. That's fine, because that's what you've decided for your soul. But if you're interested in hearing that there's another way, then throw away the devil and throw away hell.

I meet too many people who are sick and broken because they've been damaged by the dogma of a particular religion (and the food after the services!)—its doctrine of fear, anger, and sadness. I see a lot of people living in fear of something that they think is supposed to be good for them. Their minds are shackled to that tribe—the tribe of their church. And I tell them, from my own experience, "If it ain't about love, joy, and gratitude, let it go."

Now, notice I didn't say throw away all religion. I did not say throw away God. If it's a positive force in your life that doesn't hold you back, stay with it. I'm only encouraging you to beware, question everything, and throw away negativity, which is something I decided to do.

I decided I couldn't be a part of that religion anymore, because I only wanted to be part of love and joy. And I didn't like its restrictions. Despite the fact that the "Big Three" (the Abrahamic faiths of Christianity, Islam, and Judaism) have their fair share of woo-woo, they can be pretty hostile to "alternative" ideas. Personally, I found that unlocking myself from the shackles of doctrine immediately freed my mind to explore other possibilities.

## Catholic to Clairvoyant

Once I was free of religion, I started having spontaneous past-life memories. I noticed that when I met somebody, I would see something about him or her in my mind. I knew them for a reason, and I could see the story around it. I can see bits and pieces of the story, in clear pictures, as if I'm watching scenes from a movie. It's like I've clicked on the TV and there it is in glorious Technicolor. Nobody has to put me into a hypnotic state; I can spontaneously see it. I am a clairvoyant.

A clairvoyant is defined as one who sees clearly beyond what is visible to the naked eye. It can apply to seeing what is hidden in the present, what is yet to happen in the future, and what has happened in the past (recent or distant). My own special talent is seeing what is relevant to the person at the time—and what is relevant may either relate to the past or what *could happen* in the future if the current pathway does not change. (I talk more about this in the next chapter.) I can see in others their past lives, lives they are unaware they have lived. I can also see the present and future, depending on the situation. I see the people who come to me who need me to tell them something. Sometimes it's a part of their past lives; sometimes it's an issue in this life, and sometimes it's something that they will run into in the future or need to be aware of.

I'm not sure why I have this ability. At first, I was baffled, and I turned to a book by psychiatrist Dr. Brian L. Weiss, *Many Lives, Many Masters*. Weiss is a world expert in past-life regression therapy. He's an MD who has training in psychiatry. When he became a hypnotherapist, he had a client who appeared to be going into another realm under hypnosis, and gradually, he realized she was experiencing past lives. He didn't want to believe it. He was a skeptic, but he could see that her psychological condition was improving by reliving her past-life memories during the hypnosis sessions. Whatever was ailing her in this current life started to dissipate as she dealt with what had happened in her past life. This book had a profound impact on me and helped me explore my own intuitive gifts.

I learned that I could not only see other people's previous lives, but also my own. After years of piecing visions together, I now believe I am a soul that has traveled through time, and in this life, that soul has been manifested in the spirit of Veronica—me. I believe that the difference between soul and spirit is that the soul is eternal and the spirit is the personality that is embodied by various people during different lifetimes.

This is the woo-woo I'm talking about: I cannot prove anything scientifically, of course, but I know that my soul has been on a journey because I have clear past-life memories. In each of these memories, I'm looking out of the same eyes, but I know that I'm in a different body.

Let me tell you one of my most vivid recollections, which goes back to Saint Veronica. Past memories are so real and so clear for me, and they have so much emotion attached to them, that whenever I tell this story, tears well up in my eyes. I'll share some more stories from my past lives as we move forward through this book. Perhaps you're a skeptic too, just as Dr. Weiss was at first. But while at the very least, you will find them fun, I truly hope you also find them thought-provoking.

### Veronica's Veil

*I am on a dusty, primitive road. It is hard journey. It is a hot place. I am carrying a basket, picking berries on the side of the road for my family. There are lots of other people on the road, minding their own business, paying no attention to me. But there is something else happening: Men are walking along the road to their deaths.*

*It is a time in which punishments on criminals are meted out through crucifixion. Some of them are hanged upside down. I have seen this sight before. It is common to see people walking along the road carrying on their shoulders the very tree branches upon which they are to be hanged.*

As I'm picking the berries, one of the men who's carrying these branches to the site of his impending death, stops and breaks down beside me. This man, this common criminal, falls down in front of me. It is hot. He stands, picking up his branches. He is sweating.

In this society, women wear clothes that protect them from the heat, which includes wearing a veil. I take off my veil, and I wipe his brow with it. I don't have another way to help him. I feel sad for him because I know he is going to die. He lifts his branches onto his shoulders and says to me, "Keep healing the people." Then he goes on his way toward death.

I don't realize anything is amiss until later. I go home and carry on with my business. But later in the night, when I am undressing, I take off my clothes and my veil, and I realize that there's a spot in my veil, and when I look closer, I see that the spot looks like a face. As I look at it more, it looks like the face of the man I met earlier that day on the road.

The veil causes a great stir in the community, and people begin speculating about who the man could have been. My veil and I become famous. Shortly after having that experience, I decide to leave home. I am an unmarried woman in my mid-twenties (which at that time was considered too old to be single), and people know that I have a knack for being able to help people get well.

I set up a clinic with three other unmarried women. People come to our clinic as a place of last resort and for all kinds of reasons. We help them get well, and then we send them back to wherever they came from.

When we first start our clinic, we can't figure out how to make things work. I mean, we are poor. We are on the fringe of society. But one day somebody brings in a child who is very sick. We all work on him. Everyone thinks the child is going to die. The child is with us for about a week until he is completely well. We didn't know who that child was, but after he leaves our care, we start getting financial support. That support is given secretly because we are on the margins of the community and aren't widely accepted. The person who had brought the child to us must be very powerful in society because our clinic is taken care of from that moment on.

*  *  *

My church could not help me reach a greater understanding of my soul; ultimately, that understanding came from my intuition and a clairvoyant. One day I sat down with that clairvoyant for a reading. She told me, "You're a healer. You've always been a healer." What she noted is that I've been in the helping and healing profession for a lot of my "soul journey." In this life, I am a doctor, but I know from my past-life recollections that I have always been a healer of some kind. Knowing this helps me understand my calling in this life.

As an eye doctor, I've always said, "Good vision improves your outlook." Now, with the greater understanding of my gift for clairvoyance, I go further and say, "Good spiritual vision improves your outlook." We are all on a continuous soul journey, and I feel a sense of freedom in knowing that many people—including you—are experiencing this too.

**It's important that we have hope and faith, but it doesn't matter what form that faith takes, providing it is a positive force in your life and doesn't keep you shackled.**

### Gift 1: Guided Meditation

To start your journey, use this guided imagery: Meditation on Flowers at drveronica.com/flowers/

Chapter 2

# Does Your Doctor Make You Sick?

*"One of the first duties of the physician is to educate the masses not to take medicine."*
—Sir William Osler, 1849–1919,
founding professor of Johns Hopkins Hospital

It's not just institutional religion that can prevent us being well in body, mind, and spirit. The traditional medical establishment can cause us problems too. Sometimes the cure is worse than the ailment, and the statistics on hospital-acquired infections are just one of the indicators of the failure of our health care.

I was once a regular ophthalmologist. I did a year of internal medicine—a year of running around in the CCU, the ICU, and medical wards—before I went into training to become an ophthalmologist. I loved my patients but hated the way I was practicing medicine as I watched people go blind, go on dialysis, or get amputations from diseases that were avoidable. All the while, I was living a lifestyle to stay well and keep my family well, including shopping in the aisles of Whole Foods (before it was popular to do that). In my medical practice, I was using props, pills, lasers, and surgery to help people, but I never dealt with the root cause of their issues, physically or spiritually.

After months of working this way, I became clinically depressed, so one day I left. I left the practice I had started from patient zero around the same time that I left my church. I also left my husband. That all sounds pretty radical, right? Making one major change in your life can be stressful, but all those changes at once? But it wasn't radical at the time. I was called in a different direction, and I know that I would never return to that former life because it was far more stressful than the multiple changes at one time could ever have been. You might say that I saw the light! I began training in homeopathy, functional medicine, and the "woo-woo."

At this point, I'd like to share with you another of my past lives, which was first revealed to me on a visit with a talented psychic named Carol London. I went to see her after I'd left my ophthalmic practice, but before I identified as a medical intuitive. Carol took only my first name, my last name, and my birth date. With this information, she read me very accurately, telling me things about myself, my sons, my ex-husband, and the guy I was dating at the time. She knew from a friend that I was a doctor, and she asked me what kind I was. When I told her, she explained that she believed I was blind in a previous life and that I wanted to understand it. After that reading, the story began to come to me.

\* \* \*

*I am a young, attractive woman who has the ability to move energy and help people get well. I live in the Middle East, in a strict Islamic culture in which the roles of men and women and the rules of male–female interaction are clearly defined. It is very repressive for me as a young, attractive woman with talents that the men do not have.*

*One day, the men in power decide they want to use me, but not for my healing abilities. They want to use me for their desires. But they don't want me to see who they are, because they believe that if I cannot see who they are, they aren't doing anything wrong and will still be able to get into Heaven.*

*And so, one of the men puts acid drops into my eyes; they immediately cloud my corneas. I still look OK, but I can't see well. Everything becomes a blur. I can get around, but nothing has clarity and detail. There is only one face I remember well in all its detail. The face belongs to a man I love.*

## Intuition to Industrial: The Problem with Modern Medicine

People, especially here in the United States, want everything proven to them, and the FDA and the pharmaceutical industry has laid down the law on which substances and treatments are "trustworthy." The problem with that is not everything fits into science's neat little boxes. There are a lot of modalities that work but we can't explain exactly *why* they work. We know something works, and a lot of people will agree that it works, but they have no way to prove it with our current scientific knowledge.

I am an eye surgeon, a trained physician, who practices proven medical techniques. However, I am also a "medical intuitive" who also appreciates the power of "unproven" healing techniques. I keep one foot firmly planted in the orthodox and the other in the unorthodox because I see that a lot of times people are putting their faith in healthcare modalities—pharmaceuticals and surgical procedures—but these medical interventions are hurting them.

There was a time when all medicine was "woo-woo." The healers in the community were (mostly) women, who used herbal remedies and natural procedures to treat the sick. At one time, men didn't go anywhere near pregnant women. I'm over simplifying here but, in essence, female healers were pushed out of the healthcare system when the "rational" men of science decided women's approach was nothing more than hocus-pocus.

The father of homeopathy was a German named Dr. Christian Hahnemann, born in 1775. (Incidentally, there's a medical school in Philadelphia called Hahnemann University.) He was a physician who became critical of medical practices such as bloodletting, which he could see did more harm than good. One day, he observed the effect on malaria of a particular tree bark, which sparked his interest in natural remedies, and "homeopathy" was born. This took medicine back somewhat to its folk roots, and he published his first essay on homeopathy in 1796. Sometimes homeopathy is disregarded as "New Age," but there's nothing new about Hahnemann's theories, and homeopathy is still going strong more than two hundred years after Hahnemann, and it continues to grow.

The opposite of homeopathy is allopathy, which means the treatment of disease with drugs. There was a time where allopathic doctors were considered quacks! People couldn't understand the chemistry behind the powders, potions, and pills. But the allopathic doctors formed organizations, created standards, and pushed everything else aside. Eventually, allopathy pushed homeopathy to the fringe, much like the female healers were sidelined. Why? Money, probably. The female healers of days gone by weren't out to make pots of money either—it was simply part of a tradition handed down through generations—but the men who replaced them saw the potential riches to be made through chemicals and poisons. Drug companies realized that manufacturing drugs (ones that create side effects that require yet more drugs to alleviate) could generate huge wealth, and using what could be found in the forest—the freely available natural stuff—suddenly became "woo-woo."

Fast-forward to 2017, and we're all held hostage by the pharmaceutical industry. Do you know *anyone* who's not popping at least one type of pill? The TV and the Internet poke us constantly: "Are you feeling this?" "Do you suffer with that?" "Ask your doctor about such and such!"

The quote at the beginning of this chapter is from Sir William Osler, who was one of the four founding professors of Johns Hopkins Hospital. He understood the problem with prescription drugs. He said, "The person who takes medicine must recover twice, once from the disease and once from the medicine." And that's even truer today than when he was alive. The drug ads on TV spend more time telling you how bad you're going to feel taking the drug than how it's going to help you.

## Medical Intuitive: Diagnosing the Spiritual

I am now a medical intuitive reader with a functional-medicine practice. If you've never been exposed to this complement to regular healthcare practices, as many haven't, I want to explain exactly what these things are. My hope is that you decide to give functional medicine a try, not necessarily as a replacement for the health advice you get from a conventional doctor, but as a complement to it.

First, let me explain functional medicine for those of you who are new to the term. What attracted me to functional medicine is that it is not hierarchal like conventional medicine, where patients are at the mercy of the doctor's knowledge and skills. Rather, functional medicine is primarily about collaboration between the patient and the doctor: it is an empowering modality for both parties. Crucially, too, it is *proactive*, and the prevention of illness is a key concern. That is not usually true of conventional medicine! I also like functional medicine because it is rooted in science of genetics and in "real world" factors, such as the impact of environmental factors on health. And finally, functional medicine is highly personalized. When you see a functional medicine practitioner, you can be assured your treatment is all about *you*, and not the profit margins of the hospital or pharmaceutical companies. It's all about knowing what's going on in your spirit, which might be affecting your body. Alternative treatments might include traditional Chinese medicine practices, massage, reflexology, dietary supplements, physic assessment, and so on.

I practice functional medicine, and I specialize in intuitive treatments. My definition of a "medical intuitive" is someone who has strong psychic abilities, and is able to pick up information in the area of health concerns. Perhaps because of my medical training, those particular issues come through strongly for me.

Everybody defines intuitive differently. Intuitive senses are mediated in the temporal lobe of the "right brain" and there are different intuitive senses. We have five physical senses, and we have intuitive senses that mirror them:

| | |
|---|---|
| **Sight** | **Clairvoyance** is intuitive vision, which includes insightful skills such as precognition (seeing someone's past). |
| **Hearing** | **Clairaudience** is the perception of sound others cannot hear. Such sounds might travel across time. |
| **Touch** | **Clairtangency** is the ability to know something through physical touch. |
| **Taste** | **Clairgustance** is being able to taste something without it entering the mouth. |
| **Smell** | **Clairsalience** is the ability to read a person or object through fragrance that others cannot smell. |

There is also **clairsentience**, which is the ability to feel something that is intangible, such as cold temperatures, hunger, or an emotional sensation. And there is also **claircognizance,** which is an ability to suddenly know something, such as knowing who is about to call you.

We all have "clair" skills, even if we don't know it. Sometimes we can sense things without a rational explanation.

We all have these intuitive abilities, these "spider senses." We all get feelings and messages. We all have those times when we know who's on the phone or who's at the door before we answer. People who are psychic are simply able to connect more easily, and at will, with these feelings. They realize it's a skill and they develop that skill. Someone who chooses to call himself "intuitive" is simply saying that his alternative senses are stronger than the average person's. Like muscles, intuitive senses can be developed and strengthened.

I have a friend named Jayne Sanders, who is a scientific hand analyst. She can look at your hand and tell you what your master path is, your life purpose, and your unique gifts, based on the marking in your hands. This is not palm reading, but rather a scientific analysis. (There is scientific research showing that the way your brain's made is written on your hands; these are markings that you're born with, and neonatologists have studied this in infants, but it's not a widely known science as yet.) Jayne told me, "Only 10 percent of the population has any gift markings in their hand. You have eight of them. Five of them are intuitive gifts."

I use my intuitive senses to read people's energies, and because I've practiced, my ability has got better and better. Because I opened my aura and embraced the abilities that we all have, information can flow into my right brain.

Due to their sensitivity, medical intuitives are able to link spiritual and emotional issues with what's going on physically at a particular time. Often, I tell people something about what's going on in their lives that's causing a physical issue or ailment. When I read somebody intuitively, I can see a spiritual or emotional issue, and I tell him or her that there's something that must be paid attention to before physical healing is possible. Why is this important? If I see somebody is hurt, it's not enough to put a bandage on the wound; it's important to stop the bleeding.

## Seven Energies

Readings are all about energy centers. Again, we all know about energies because we all know people whom we consider to be "high energy" or "low energy." Or you may meet somebody and have an instant strong dislike for him or her, or feel an immediate affinity. You might really just want to be around that individual or leave his or her space as quickly as possible. Why is that? I believe that we are all set to a particular frequency, and we tend to gravitate toward people who are on a similar frequency. As human beings, we are drawn to higher frequencies of people and of emotions. Sadness is a very low frequency (low energy) and joy is high frequency (high energy). There's a great book by David R. Hawkins called *Power vs. Force* that will help you understand this in more detail if you're interested in doing so.

So, how does energy flow around our bodies? The Ayurvedic system, which comes from India, identifies "energy centers." If you do yoga, you might know the energy centers as "chakras."

The seven energy centers are located all over the body, and those energy centers have physical, emotional, and spiritual links.

A reading can work out a physical problem by first identifying a "blocked" chakra, or a reading can work backwards, meaning that it's possible to identify a problem in a particular energy center based on the ailment.

## What to Expect of a Reading

Each medical intuitive practitioner has a different methodology, but let me tell you how I operate.

When I do a reading, I just ask for the client's name, age, and gender. And then I do the reading without even meeting him or her; I'm tapping into his or her energy over time and space.

As I mentioned earlier, when I do a reading, I see what is relevant to that person at the time of the reading—something in his or her current lifetime, or something from a past life, or something that *could happen* in that individual's future if the current pathway is not changed. This is not the same as fortune-telling. Fortune-tellers take away your power by giving you a vision of an inevitable future, whereas my kind of intuitive reading provides you with the tools to take control of your own future.

I never tell people too many specific details about a medical problem I can see because it might become a self-fulfilling prophecy, meaning that the patient might become fixated on that diagnosis. As with conventional medicine, diagnoses can turn out to be incorrect (or not the full picture), and I don't want to put someone on a path that may be wrong for them or that opens me up to litigation (our rational-based legal system is not known for giving proper credence to woo-woo!). In my readings, I provide patients with sufficient information to set them on the path to an accurate diagnosis from their conventional medical team.

My training in conventional medicine works into my readings. I can identify problems from a physical standpoint and identify the emotional cause, but I don't pretend to know everything. Sometimes people need more than I can offer, so I might refer them to other practitioners. I tend to get frustrated with clients who rely too heavily on spiritual and emotional problems when there are clearly physical problems that need to be urgently addressed. I see too many people who seek out spiritual and alternative solutions and say, "Look! I'm working on myself! I'm working on myself!" but they are neglecting the physical stuff. They definitely need to work on that physical stuff, however, because once you take care of the physical, it allows more bandwidth to work on the spiritual and emotional.

What happens a lot times is I'll receive a download containing information about what clients should to do to address their health problems. Can it be tested and verified by science? Sometimes, yes; sometimes, no. It comes down to having faith in the process and the physician. It's my ultimate goal to help my clients improve their health.

I think it's fun to see information about people, of course, but I provide it as a service, because I want people to have good information that enables them to change. I can switch on my science background to be able to help people when their body is breaking down. It's important to me to use the conventional and the alternative together. Unfortunately, regular doctors don't do the same. When you see a doctor and ask a question, don't expect a spiritual answer along with the physical answer!

When the reading is done, my client and I have a question-and-answer session. Somebody may ask me about a particular relationship they're in, for example, and as soon as she asks a specific question, she opens herself up, and I'm able to see into her system. My strongest intuitive sense is clairvoyance, and I see stories play out like movie scenes.

Of course, I charge for my service, but I want people to trust me, so I provide a "try before you buy" option. I tell the client, "I'm going to read you for five minutes. If you like and believe what I'm saying, and it resonates with you, we keep going. If it's not resonating and I'm completely off base, I will give you all your money back." I want to do what I do in an ethical way. If, for whatever reason, I cannot get a reading on a person, I'll tell him so and give him his money back. It's not my goal to string people along; it's my goal to provide them with really deep, useful knowledge.

What a medical intuitive isn't is a human CAT scan machine, so don't visit a reader for an exact diagnosis. It's important for me to reiterate that what I practice is *complementary* medicine that works in conjunction with conventional medicine. I make sure that all my clients know that readings are not 100 percent accurate; they are usually about 75 percent accurate. But this is no worse than conventional medicine. To quote our friend Sir William Osler again, "Medicine is a science of uncertainty and an art of probability."

It's hard to turn off my psychic abilities, and I often find myself doing informal readings when I'm going about my regular activities. There was a woman at my gym about whom I used to receive overwhelming messages regarding a drug addiction. But I don't necessarily tell people that they have an issue. When they don't ask for the information, they're not necessarily open to hearing it. When I get a serious message, however, I will sometimes ask the person if he or she is open to hearing it.

Over the years, I have learned to identify the messages I receive from ascended masters (people who are outside of this realm) who help trained psychics notice this type of information.

## Finding a Medical Intuitive

I think locating a medical intuitive is a challenge for people who have never been down this road before because there are no "standards" or regulations, as there are in conventional medicine. If you're looking for somebody to help you with your health specifically, try to find someone with a good medical background. I know there are good psychics out there providing a lot of good information, but many of them cannot enable you to determine how to solve a physical problem. There are also many frauds in the psychic field, but the same is true of any industry you can think of, so do your research.

**Science can take us only so far with the body. If you're serious about your health, you must take care of your spiritual and emotional wellbeing. By combining conventional and alternative treatments, you can treat your body, your mind, and your soul.**

## Gift 2: Discover Your Toxicity

Many people are exposed to stress and toxins. There are three types of toxic stress: physical, chemical, and emotional. Take this "Are You Toxic?" quiz about physical and chemical toxins to find out your risk level:

drveronica.wufoo.com/forms/are-you-toxic/

## Chapter 3
# Miracles (Bending the Rules)

*"Change your perception of what a miracle is, and you'll see them all around you."*
—Jon Bon Jovi, American singer-songwriter, activist, and philanthropist

Miraculous recoveries from serious illnesses happen. When someone defies the odds of survival, the scientific minded will claim there is a rational explanation that medicine simply hasn't discovered yet, and the religious minded will attribute the recovery to the power of faith and divine grace.

I've heard a miracle described as "God bending the rules." From a medical standpoint, that could be translated to "science bending the rules." But I think that treating miracles as inexplicable—whether from a scientific or a religious standpoint—is damaging: it denies us the power we have over ourselves as individuals.

I believe miracles happen when *we* bend *our own* rules. People make miracles possible when they shift their thinking and open themselves up to something that yesterday seemed impossible. The simple change of mindset is, for me, a kind of miracle. It's what enables someone who is three hundred pounds to drop so much weight that she ends up comfortable wearing a bikini. This isn't God or science bending the rules; it's the individual who's bending the rules by which she had been living—rules that she may have set for herself or those set for her by others. These individuals defy their own expectations by deciding to go with the flow of their unique body, mind, and spirit.

Let's say someone has cancer. One test shows cancer, but the next round of tests is negative. That's miraculous, because it defied what was known about the situation. Do things like that happen? Yes, they do. But I believe they occur because somebody made such a change in his emotional and spiritual state, and had so much faith in himself that he could beat the cancer.

In Part Two of this book, we'll discuss in more depth how thinking differently can help us heal, but for now, I'd like to share another of my woo-woo stories. It's not so much a story about health as it is a story about the heart. It's an account of

## Miracles (Bending the Rules)

a romantic miracle in my own life that shows the power of mind over matter.

* * *

It's October 2010. I visit a psychic for a reading and she tells me I'm going to get married in 2012. I think, This woman's way off! I'm dating some guys, but the relationships are nothing very serious. The year 2012 isn't too far off. How am I going to meet somebody, fall in love, and become comfortable enough with him to marry him the year after next? The rest of the reading is good, but I disregard this particular insight and soon forget it.

On Christmas Eve 2010, I attend a friend's party. Leo is the only black guy I've met in my small, very white town, so we become friends easily. I had stayed in the town after my divorce, but there was no logical reason for me to have done so. Maybe I'd stayed local because I knew deep down that I needed to meet my future husband?

Leo and I meet in the local store, which Leo owns. He is incredibly cosmopolitan and fascinating, and we like each other—though not on a romantic level, just as friends. I feel like he's my brother.

I don't want to go to his Christmas Eve party because I don't want to attend as a single woman. I'm tired of going places as a single woman. However, for some reason, I don't back out; l go.

Leo introduces me to the people in the room. I say hi to all the guys, purposefully not engaging much with them because I assume most are married, and I don't want the women to think I'm trying to hit on their husbands. I say hello to be polite, and I move on.

I am on the outside of the group. Leo, his family, and many of his friends are from French-speaking Africa, and I don't speak French. However, Leo's wife and some other party attendees are American, so I end up talking to these individuals with whom I have more in common despite the fact that they're mostly white.

Dinnertime arrives. I survey the spread of traditional African foods, which are very different from what Americans eat.

A guy walks up to me and says, "You should taste that right there." It is some type of shredded meat.

I don't turn to look at him; I simply reply, "Thank you. I'll try it."

I am counting down the time until I can politely leave, thinking, I came. I put in my time. I was polite and nice. Now it's time to go home. Who wants to be the only single person at a party?

In early January 2011, I am talking with Leo. I say, "You've got to have one single friend, somebody to whom you can introduce me."

He replies, "I do. You met him at my party."

"Everyone was married," I say.

Leo shakes his head and tells me about the guy I had met at the table. "His name is Abel. He's a Tae Kwon Do master, and he's really fit."

## Miracles (Bending the Rules)

*Leo gets Abel on the phone right away, and I start talking to him. We have a nice conversation. I tell him I'm a Tae Kwon Do black belt (which I am), and he's impressed. He's also impressed I'm an eye doctor because he needs his vision checked! He says that we should meet next time I'm in New York, which is where he lives. There is no big plan. We text a couple times after that and talk on the phone a few times.*

*One day, during one of our phone calls, he says, "I just want to let you know, before anything starts, that I'm not really interested in getting married. I just want to be very honest with you and open with you up front."*

*I don't care. I've been married before. I really don't want to get married.*

*So I say, "That's totally cool. I've done marriage and the white, picket-fence life. Nothing is real until it is real."*

*We agree that if we see each other, fine; we'll just go with the flow.*

*I call him a few days before January 20—my birthday—and say, "I'm coming to New York to celebrate with a few friends. Are you available?"*

*He is, and we agree to meet at my hotel in Times Square.*

*He comes to the hotel and says, "I'm here," and I go downstairs to meet him, but I have no idea what he looks like. I'm on a blind date! Then I see someone who I know is Abel.*

## But Now I See

*We end up going to the restaurant and talking. I'm having dinner with him and thinking,* This guy is really cool. I like him. *By the end of the night, I am thinking,* He's a keeper! *I'm not considering the possibility of marriage because this is our first date, but I'd like to keep him on the roster of guys I'm dating!*

*A little while after, I invite him to visit me. We have another great night together and, this time, he stays over. In the middle of the night I wake up. I see him sleeping and say to myself,* He belongs in my bed. He just looks so perfect there. That's his spot.

*One day, not long into our relationship, he says, "I think you're the one. I'm going to make you my wife."*

*I'm surprised.*

*"Well, wait a second," I say. "You said you never wanted to get married. Nothing's real until it's real."*

*I refuse to believe he is serious until that June, when he asks me to marry him. I am caught off guard. I genuinely hadn't thought he was serious about wanting to make me his wife. But I say yes, and we set a date for December 31, 2011.*

* * *

You might say, "2011? The reading was wrong!" However, it was New Year's Eve and we knew it would be 2012 somewhere on Earth at the time we got married, so the reading was right

## Miracles (Bending the Rules)

enough for me. Later, it transpired that the reading was right more than once. My husband is Catholic, and having jumped all the hoops the church set up for us to have the Catholic wedding my husband wanted, we were finally married in the eyes of God (according to the Catholic Church) in March 2012. We even had an extra Catholic ceremony in France in June 2012. So, my psychic reading wasn't correct once, but rather, *three* times!

Now, was this a miracle? By my definition, absolutely. The marriage was miraculous because I had shifted my thinking. I had gone from never wanting to remarry to wanting to find a true soulmate. The shift had taken place when I read a book called *The Soulmate Secret*, by Arielle Ford, whom I had interviewed on my radio show. The premise of *The Soulmate Secret* is that you can script your life in such a way as to enable your soul mate to enter it. That includes making physical space (your closet or garage, perhaps), as well as time in your life for your potential soulmate. I had done all that because I wanted a partner. Marriage wasn't necessarily the endgame; my goal was simply to meet my perfect partner.

**Focus your mind and the rest will follow. You have the power to bring about miracles in your life and your health by opening your mind, your heart, and your spirit to the possibilities.**

### Gift 3: Personalized Meditation

We are all unique beings, and so guidance on health issues must also be unique. My third gift to you is a 50 percent discount on a personalized Health Creation Meditation:

drveronica.wufoo.com/forms/
special-offer-health-creation-meditation/

*Part Two*
# Get with the You-You

*"Give to yourself as much as you give of yourself!
This means you have to put yourself first."*
—Suze Orman, American author

In Part One, I explained the woo-woo. It was important for me to lay out the complementary, alternative ways of thinking about your life and health before we zero in on *you*. Hopefully, you didn't throw the book across the room, and you're still with me for Part Two!

Taking what we've learned about woo-woo, in this section of the book, we will look at how you can refocus on your spirit, your mind, and your body—in that order. This part is all about the "you-you"!

Chapter 4

# Your Spirit

I've met many people who are afraid of dying. It's understandable. But the reality is this: the moment you're born, you begin to die. We interpret death as something bad, but death just means that you've reached the end of your time in *this* life.

I can tell you from my studies, reading, and my own intuitive knowledge that this life *isn't* all there is. It's just where you are right now. You're here to learn a lesson, and your soul is on a continuous journey through time and space. You've been here before and you're going to be here again. You're a ball of energy, and science tells us that energy can never disappear; it can only transform.

When you open your mind and realize that you're spirit is an energy that *has* always been and *will* always be, death goes from being a scary prospect to an exciting one. Who will I be next? Where will I live? Freeing yourself of the fear of death in this life will enable you to live it in a healthier manner.

I believe that every living thing is on a continuous spiritual journey. Take my two dogs, for example. My dogs are in this life with me as companions, as they have been in my previous lives as well. In one of my previous lives, they weren't dogs; they were peacocks. One was a male peacock and one was a female. They were given to my husband and I as a wedding gift. We were a regal couple and the gifts came to us from another powerful couple. I'm talking about Egypt in the time before Christ, but I'm not joking when I tell you that I met that couple again in this life! I was at a past-life-regression conference when I met the couple, and I told them the story. When I'd finished, the woman said to me that she'd told her partner earlier that she thought I looked like someone. Amusingly, that someone turned out to be the African queen in Michael Jackson's video for his song "Remember the Time." But funnier still was the fact that, some time before, when she had first realized she was in love with the man, she had given him a greeting card with a peacock on it! She actually had that card with her that day and showed it to me!

Here's another story: Remember my tale about being blinded in a previous life by men who wanted only to use me for sex? Well, in 2015, I was at a conference and dropped by a booth in the exhibit hall to say hello to a woman I knew. I met a man at the booth who I also knew, but not in this life. I recognized him instantly as the soul I had known in that past life, my blind life. He was the man whom I'd loved. Because I'm not exactly the shy, retiring type, I told him that I knew him.

When I meet people this way, I always ask them, "Would you like to know something about your life?" This is because I know that I'm telling them for a particular reason, which I am not always aware of myself. The man was interested and I told him a little bit about the story. I don't go into much detail because if it resonates with that person, he or she will be able to fill in the details on his or her own.

This particular man listened and thanked me for telling him. Maybe he thought I was crazy or maybe he didn't; I don't care! It's my calling to tell people the information that comes to me, and it's their responsibility to determine what that information means to them.

## Spiritual Evaluation: Asking Deeper Questions

Everyone should get into the habit of conducting spiritual self-evaluation. Why? Because we can't expect that others will understand us if we do not fully understand ourselves.

You should never *have* to rely on a psychic or medical intuitive for insights into your soul, your mind, or your body. It's not a good thing when people become too dependent on any type of healer. They are the hypochondriacs that all medical practitioners—conventional or complementary—dread! I don't say that to be unkind; it's just that physicians find hypochondriacs very difficult to treat. Mostly, hypochondria stems from fear that can be buried deep in the psyche. Treating a hypochondriac is like playing an endless game of Whac-A-Mole; you beat one thing down and two other things pop up!

There is a big movement for "patient rights." Patients certainly do have rights and they are encouraged to exercise them, but that doesn't mean that patients should always pressure their healthcare providers. For me, the kind of power you should have is the power that comes from understanding that the choices *you* make in life create your circumstances. It is the lifestyle choices you've made—either in this life or in other lives—that lead to sickness and disease. Of course, nobody deliberately chooses to have cancer, diabetes, high blood pressure, high cholesterol, fibromyalgia, or thyroid disease! My point is that we make choices that have side effects. Here's a simple example: A study by Public Health Ontario, published in the *Lancet* medical journal in January 2017, showed that living close to a major road can increase a person's chances of developing dementia later on by 12 percent.[1] Now, we instinctively know that breathing in vehicle fumes is bad for us, so why would we

---

[1] "Living near major roads and the incidence of dementia, Parkinson's disease, and multiple sclerosis: a population-based cohort study," *The Lancet*, Vol 389, No. 10070, p718–726, 18 February 2017. DOI: http://dx.doi.org/10.1016/S0140-6736(16)32399-6

expose ourselves to it day after day? A more obvious example is that we know too much sugar makes us fat and gives us diabetes, yet we (as a nation) continue to get fatter and sicker.

I believe that the only way to gain the right kind of patient "power" is to understand the choices we make as people, and the only way to do that is by spiritual self-evaluation.

We should know ourselves spiritually because we must all try to be as self-sufficient as possible. But, if you do decide you need a little extra help in determining what's going on with you—as we all do from time to time—wouldn't it be nice to talk to a medical intuitive or clairvoyant from a place of self-awareness?

## Build Your Self-Evaluation Skills

When it comes to self-evaluation, people say, "I can't do that." They are so removed from their own spirituality that self-evaluation is too abstract, but it's possible to learn how to do it. New skills take patience and practice, but they will come if you apply some commitment. If you want to create a successful self-evaluation process, you must quiet the voices in your head that say, "No, I can't; I'm not capable."

### Step One: Experience

If you do the same thing every day, you don't necessarily grow and learn spiritually because you're not having a full spectrum of experiences. Let's say you're a part of a particular religion and you enjoy it. Have you ever stepped outside of it for a moment to experience other people's belief systems? I'm not suggesting you convert from Christianity to Judaism, for example, just that you broaden your awareness of different faiths. It may bring your own faith into sharper focus or it may lead you to question aspects of it. It can give you a different perspective in learning and respecting that everybody is on a different journey.

Even bad experiences are good. If you have had something very traumatic happen in your life and you've come out the other end, you can learn from it.

### Step Two: Observe

If you visit another place of worship (preferably belonging to a religion different from the one you're used to), for example, observe what's going on around you. Just take it in without judgment. Make a mental note of how you feel. *I feel happy/confused/furious/calm.* Or write down your observations and impressions in a journal afterward: what you saw, what you thought, what you smelled, what you heard, the people who made an impact, what surprised you the most, what was similar to your own practice, and what was different from your own practice. Write down anything that you think may help you grow and evolve.

Ask yourself some questions about the experience. Don't worry about answering them right away. No question is too big; no question is too small. Little kids constantly ask *why*. They ask it about things we think are so obvious. It's "why this," "why that" all the time. That's the place to which you need to return.

"Why did I meet that person today?" "Why did we have that conversation?" If somebody enters your world for only five minutes and says something to you that stays with you, ask yourself why it was interesting. In my experience, it doesn't always have to be somebody I know. It might be the guy who put me in a taxi at a hotel. Spiritual evaluation is asking yourself the deeper questions. But asking the question is the first step; next, you have to find an answer, and for that, you need to make some quiet time.

### Step Three: Meditation

Meditation is about setting aside time for *you*. Time for you is not necessarily about pampering yourself—though a spa can be a great place to have time to yourself; it's about having enough time to relax and put things into perspective so that emotions aren't swinging around all the time.

Meditation is about being able to think clearly with no distractions. You have to learn to start being alone: no TV, no radio, no anything. Just *be*. It's incredibly hard to find a place and time in our busy lives for solitude, but it's so important.

Now, everyone meditates differently. There's no one right way, necessarily. You don't have to sit cross-legged; you don't have to meditate for a particular length of time. Me? I work out as much as I can and hard as I can. Then, after that, I'm so tired that all I literally can't do anything else, so my mind is clear enough to meditate.

If you struggle to find time, join a basic yoga class. All yoga classes should have meditation time built into them. The movement part of yoga is good exercise, but the original purpose of yoga was to balance your body so that you can meditate better. There's also a focus on breathing, which can help clear your mind of other things.

Yoga can help you clear your mind, but the objective of the meditation I'm talking about is not about thinking about nothing; the purpose is to think about yourself. What do you need? How do you feel physically and emotionally? Why did you react that way to that problem at work or at home?

Spiritual evaluation doesn't require more than your own introspection. But in order to have that introspection, you've got to make some time. You have to relax, even if you are the type of person who doesn't like to be alone. Perhaps you always have to have the TV or radio on. If you're the type who always has to be doing something, really ask yourself why. Ask yourself what you think is going to happen to you if you're alone for a while. Find the cord and follow it back to the origin of the fear.

### Step Four: Action

Spiritual evaluation gets you to a point of greater understanding, but that's where most people stop. You've asked the question and found an answer within yourself. So what now? Don't leave a problem unsolved! Seek help from people who can help you deal with it if it's something that's holding you back in body, mind, or spirit.

Sometimes there is a role for someone else to play in your self-evaluation, and this is not necessarily a religious leader or a guru. It might just be someone you can rely on to ask you some tough questions. We all need somebody who will help us think sometimes.

This is particularly true when a traumatic or abusive situation is involved. Those are the hardest situations to experience and observe or on which to meditate. For me, that situation was divorce, which is traumatic for a lot of people. But what does one learn from that? Not that the other person was a jerk or whatever—even if the other person really *was* a jerk—but why you ended up in that relationship in the first place. What part did you play? What choices did you make that brought about the trauma?

Now that you know the steps, try to make time each day for self-evaluation; with time, it will hopefully become a habit.

## Spiritual Amnesia

We're born into this life to particular parents who taught us what we're supposed to think and feel. Society also teaches you what you're supposed to think and feel.

I've been brought into this life as an African-American woman. I've had different cultures and traditions passed on to me by my parents. They did the best they knew how, as does everybody. However, just because my parents raised me a certain way, it doesn't mean that they got it absolutely right. We all have to start acknowledging and questioning everything we know of the world and ourselves through evaluation of our own spirit.

While you're on your soul journey, you enter each new life with amnesia. This is the way the universe is made, so it's not your fault. We all signed on to receive this amnesia as babies, and to have our soul evolve through a particular life. What do I mean by "signed on to"? I believe that we select what experiences and lessons we would like to have before we are born. Then, before we arrive in this life, we make agreements with other souls who will help us have those experiences and learn those lessons. It's a strange idea for some, perhaps, that we choose our lives and that nothing is random. I choose not to believe we are victims of circumstance. I knew what my soul needed to learn before I entered into this life, and I collude with other souls so that my spiritual growth can continue.

This belief developed when I read the work of Dr. Michael Newton, a psychologist who talks about the soul journey, the soul between the lives—not what happens in past lives, but what happens *between* past lives. It is during this time between lives that we plan for the life to come and identify the mentors and masters from whom we will learn. This was a life-changing revelation for me because it made me see that we're all on a continuum. When I realized that I wasn't crazy and that other people are experiencing the same phenomena in their lives, it gave me power. It also made me happy to know that our souls are evolving and on a never-ending journey. In each life, we're here to learn and complete a particular project or path—maybe *many* projects and paths.

Unless you're naturally intuitive, you don't remember what happened before you were born into this life. I'm one of those people who have memories of that time, but for many years, I couldn't figure out what these memories—these flashes and flickers—were. I couldn't unscramble them for myself, and I couldn't ask questions because the people surrounding me weren't people I could talk to about it. During this period, I discovered some of the most life-changing works that I've ever read, in particular, Dr. Brian L. Weiss' first book, *Many Lives, Many Masters*. As I mentioned in Chapter 1, Dr. Weiss is a world expert in past-life regression therapy.

Through reading about the subject, I discovered that if you explore yourself spiritually, you can begin to shed some of the amnesia you're born with, and when you open up to the possibilities of the past and the future, you'll understand how to heal yourself.

## Spiritual Self-Diagnosis

When you're sick, that's a sign from the universe, saying, "You've gotta do something about X or Y." Let's take a serious example.

When a woman has breast cancer, it's not just because she has a BRCA gene; it's that the BRCA gene is switched on. We know that genes get turned on and off. It could be environmental or it could relate to lifestyle, but it also can be related to stress. And that stress can be emotional or spiritual.

One day, during a course I was taking on homeopathy, I happened to sit down with a woman and her adult daughter for lunch. They were members of my class, and I had never met them before; they were visiting from another section of the class for that day only. I noted the woman when I entered the room because she had bruises around her left eye. It looked like an old injury, but I didn't want to assume anything, so I did not ask any questions. During lunch, I explained to them what I do as a medical intuitive and how emotional and spiritual stress is linked to illnesses and injuries.

I said, "For example, let's think about a woman who has breast cancer."

I then talked about the difficulties women suffering from breast cancer can face in their relationships and also how they can feel about themselves. Oftentimes, women do not like themselves, believing they're not good enough and feeling

## Your Spirit

unhappy with some of their relationships. When I finished talking, the woman and her daughter looked at each other.

The woman said, "I'm a two-time breast-cancer survivor, and I've been in a very abusive relationship."

That's getting an intuitive hit! I didn't know anything about that woman, but I was able to read into her story and show her the possibility that the abusive relationship was a stress trigger that the cancer needed to grow. She needed to hear that message, but what she would do with that information was up to her.

Everything is up to you. You are in control of your body, mind, and spirit. I only help people explore their soul so that they can reach their own spiritual diagnosis. I cannot be the healer, only the messenger. Ultimately, people heal themselves; therefore, when people engage me, I simply give them as many messages as I can. Whenever you're getting a message, you need to stand up, pay attention, and think about why you're receiving that message. Getting a message is a sign you're on the wrong pathway and that you should turn around or go get help.

**By being more spiritually self-aware, you will more readily recognize when you're being given messages about your wellbeing, and you'll be able to self-diagnose your problems with more accuracy.**

### Gift 4: Half-Price Intuitive Reading

Although it is fascinating in its own right, medical intuition has a purpose. It is my aim in this book to guide you toward confronting difficult issues, but only an intuitive reading can provide suggestions on what your unique energetic aura is asking for. Exclusively to my readers, I am offering a half-price intuitive reading—a gift worth up to $500! Claim your half-price reading here: drveronica.wufoo.com/forms/special-offer-full-medical-intuitive-reading/

Chapter 5

# Your Mind

*"We are shaped by our thoughts;
we become what we think. When the mind is pure,
joy follows like a shadow that never leaves."*
—Buddha

Our spirits are an overarching universal force—an essence, an energy. And whether we give off positive or negative energy depends very much on our mental health. Even if you don't care about your spiritual energy, you know instinctively that poor mental health can, at best, zap your bodily energy and, at worst, make you seriously ill. Yet too often we neglect the state of our minds, or we actively continue practicing bad behaviors and habits that worsen the situation.

This thing we call "life" isn't all fun and games. Life can be one challenge after another. The people who live long and live well are the people who know how to overcome these challenges—and sometimes even avoid the challenges in the first place. As you overcome your challenges, whether they be emotional or physical, mastering your mind is how you will move forward in life and continue your spiritual journey.

## Eight Easy Ways to Stay Sane

Here are some ways you can take care of your mental wellbeing without paying a dime.

### Method One: Owning It
### (It's Not Them; It's You)

There's a lot of blame going around. When something happens to someone that he or she interprets as negative, there can be a lot of finger pointing. Most of the time, the finger is pointing at somebody who's close to you when it ought to be pointed to yourself. "But, Dr. Veronica, it was her fault! She made me feel this way!" No. Wrong.

When you feel stressed and unhappy, it's not your wife; it's not your mother, father, sister, or brother. It's not the government that is causing you stress. It's not the wars on the other side of the world that are causing you stress. It is *you* who is causing you the stress. How you interpret life is your responsibility. You can interpret it in a positive sense, a negative sense, or a neutral sense.

The Buddhist philosophy is that everything just *is*. It's not good. It's not bad. It just is. The people who get to the

## Your Mind

point where they can say, "It just is. This is our challenge in the world. This is what life is all about," are the people who are able to realize that they have control over their emotions.

The control of your emotions and your spirit is where you get your power. Those who point the finger are victims. The victims get sick and they have all manners of horrible things happen to them, and they say, "This is horrible. Life is horrible."

The people who know how to win at life are the people who point the finger at themselves and realize that they can interpret a situation however they want to. By choosing to interpret the situation in a way that helps you make some sense of it, you are choosing the healthiest option for your spirit and body: "This is a lesson. There's something bad happening, but it's a lesson for me, and therefore, it's good. I was allowed to have this lesson, and I'm going to move on."

There's been a lot made about the power of positive thinking, but we never really understood until recently how much that thinking changes our physiology. There's a great book I recommend to all of my clients: *The Biology of Belief*, by Dr. Bruce H. Lipton.

Lipton is a microbiologist, and he has shown that how you think changes your cellular physiology. So it's quite important for you to realize that whether you're thinking positively or negatively, your cellular physiology is changing. When you're thinking positively, you *feel* good. When there's something that causes you to think negatively, when you translate emotions into some form of fear, anger, or sadness, you are self-harming on the cellular level. I'm making this very simple at this point: When you're in a state of love and joy, your cells are healthier and can more easily fend off illness and of injury. When you're in constant state of fear, anger, and sadness, your body is much more prone to sickness.

### Method Two: *Altitude* of Gratitude

No, that's not a misspelling. Gratitude is an attitude, but it's also a higher form of emotion.

As I pointed out in an earlier chapter, everything (from color to sound to objects) has an energy, and that energy is given off in vibrations. Different thoughts, different feelings, and different attitudes have particular vibrations. Different levels of energy have an effect on our bodies.

Most people think the highest level of vibration is love. Although love is pretty high up there and can change a person's physical wellbeing a lot, in fact, the highest level of vibration is gratitude. Some people call it the "attitude of gratitude," but I call it the "altitude of gratitude" because it's so high up there.

In the King James Bible, Philippians 4:11, Paul says, "Not that I speak in respect of want: for I have learned, in whatsoever state I am, *therewith* to be content." That's what we should all strive for. Even when terrible things happen, we should be saying, "Thank you for allowing this to happen to me." It's not easy. In fact, next to forgiveness, gratitude is one of the hardest skills to master. But trust me and try it. All of the sudden, your body will shift. Your soul will shift.

It's really easy to be happy and to be grateful when everything is good. But the altitude of gratitude will help you keep your head above water when you're really put to the test, when life is throwing things at you and you're in the crucible, being ground down. When life threatens to overwhelm you, you have to fly up, up, and away into your higher spiritual plane. Look down at what's going on and believe, "I know something amazing is going to happen soon. The only reason I would go through this dark tunnel is because there's something wonderful on the other side, and I'm happy and grateful about that."

## Method Three: Love What You See in the Mirror

Some people think that if you love yourself, your ego is too big—and, of course, there is such a thing as narcissism. Narcissists suck all of the air out of the room, and they can only talk about themselves. We all know them when we meet them. I'm not talking about a pathological love of yourself here, a self-love that hurts everybody else around you. Rather, I'm talking about feeling good about yourself—realizing that you are a unique individual, and that as a unique individual, you're a part of the creation and linked to everything else that is created. When you love yourself, there's no inside, and there's no outside.

One of the ways in which many people mess up supremely in life is in their choice of romantic partners. There are many people—both men and women—who repeatedly select partners who treat them like crap. Ultimately, this is because these individuals feel bad about themselves.

You have to realize that you can only be well in body, mind, and spirit if you love yourself. When you love yourself, you will attract partners who will love you just as much. It is important to your spirit and mind to be with people who are kind and loving.

You know that love and joy are healing emotions that keep you healthy. The fear, anger, and sadness—the drama in your relationships—are negative and self-harming. In the same way that you would never knowingly ingest poison or rotten food, don't let toxic love into your body. That man you keep going back to despite his ill-treatment of you, or that woman you just can't get enough of, might be the cause of stress that could damage the health of your body. Sex with someone who's not right for you might feel good in the moment, but sex is the act of sharing the temple of your body with someone. It's your temple; don't let in the philistines! They will only make you feel bad about yourself when the moment is over, and that will infect your sense of self. Remember, self-loathing is a sexually transmitted disease!

If you find yourself wondering either, "Why do I always attract jerks?" or "Why do I always pick the pretty girl who's a bitch to me?" it's because you're not loving yourself properly. You need to really look at the soul of the person you're with, because whatever you're seeing there is what's in *you*. Realize that you're looking into a mirror.

Let me tell you about a condition that I have named the "Janay Rice Syndrome." In case you don't know Janay's story, here's a summary: Janay believed that being knocked around by her husband—the former Baltimore Ravens player Ray Rice—was God's way of raising the public's awareness of domestic violence. But my question is: What was it within Janay that led her to feel she deserved to be abused? The "Janay Rice Syndrome" is what I call the situation people get into of attracting crap in their life because they feel like crap. Crap attracts crap! I tell my patients often, "If you feel bad about yourself, bad things will surely happen to you."

In the 1930s, there was an experiment conducted on monkeys that resulted in the discovery of what was called "Klüver-Bucy syndrome," named after the two researchers. The monkeys were given brain lesions that made them irresistibly attracted to dangerous predators. Over time, instead of running from obvious danger, these monkeys ran *toward* their natural predators; they couldn't help themselves. Similarly, I believe certain people are drawn to predatory relationships because of their own psychological trauma and drama. They can't help themselves and believe they are destined to love these poisonous people because they can't do anything else. "He didn't really mean to beat me up and make me pass out. You're not being fair to him!" Like the monkeys with their brain lesions, these people's brains have been rewired by trauma so that they are drawn to the fear, anger, and sadness these relationships bring.

If you often make poor romantic choices, there's only one way to get over it: have someone else pick your dates! Seriously. Get a *close* friend who loves you and knows you to set you up with someone. A true friend won't pick someone bad for you. In this way, you can learn new habits and how to appreciate the right kind of person. Turn over your love life to someone who can objectively steer you toward those who are good for you, and *away* from the Ray Rices of the world.

The secret to being loved is learning to love better, which means thinking of everything as having a cloak of love wrapped around it, and continuously asking, "How do I do this in the most loving way possible?" But that does not mean being a doormat and an enabler, like Janay Rice! Being an enabler is not being the best lover you can possibly be. There is something called "tough love," and sometimes you have to have to employ it.

Ultimately, what you need to remember with romantic love is that you have to care for yourself first. When you do so, you can expect to be treated right by the romantic partners who come into your life. Therefore, my advice to you is: stop sleeping with the devil!

## Your Mind

### Method Four: Stay in Good Company

As an entrepreneur, I've gone to many conferences at which I've heard, "Your network is your net worth." The same can be applied to your spiritual life.

You must understand that the company you keep is of the utmost importance. It says everything about you—not just how much money you're going to have, because that isn't the most important thing in life, but whether you're going to be well or sick.

Some studies have shown that people with good, sizeable social networks live longer. Loneliness literally kills. But more than that, the "birds of a feather" phenomenon applies to your network. Studies show that friends even tend to be of a similar size! Fat people get fatter together, and skinny people get skinnier together.

Realize that whom you're hanging out with is of utmost importance to your health. If you desire good health, choose to spend your time with other people who desire good health—those who possess values similar to your own and who think of their body as their temple.

The brutal truth is that if you would like to be healthier, you have to pick better friends. If your family has lots of health problems, you have to find an additional family with which to spend time. Some people buy into the notion that they have particular diseases because it runs in their family. But epigenetics now tells us that DNA—what runs in the family—is approximately only 25 percent of the story. That means that the other 75 percent is within your control. Families tend to pass down not only genetics, but also a spiritual journey, a way of looking at the world, a way of talking, thinking, acting, and eating. If yours is a beautiful family of peacocks that has given you a positive outlook and high energy, great! If your family is a kettle of scavenging vultures, you're going to need to find a new flock of birds with brighter plumage!

Maybe your current circle of friends and family are just fine, but there's something missing. If that is the case, seek out new people who have the personality traits that you would like to develop. If you come across people who have the kind of spiritual life that you would like to lead, get to know them. If you find people who have the kind of health you would like to have, find a way to become closer to them.

Of course, this all relates to the objective of loving yourself. Just as you should refuse to spend time with lovers who don't reflect the love you have for yourself, so should you refuse to be around people who do not hold similar values, and that includes family and friends. You must get to the point where you love yourself enough that you surround yourself with individuals who are beneficial to your health from an emotional and spiritual standpoint. In order to to be able to draw the healthiest people to you, you have to walk in the confidence of self-love.

### Method Five: Go off the Grid (Or, at Least, Turn off the News!)

You might have noticed that some of the healthiest people are people who have developed what's called "detachment." This is a concept that has not taken off in a big way in American society, but it's a good idea. Detachment doesn't mean you don't care about people; it doesn't mean you don't love people. It's just that you say, "This is not good, but it also isn't bad. It just *is*."

Someone who has mastered the skill of detachment can watch Fox News or CNN without bursting a blood vessel. A detached person can flip back and forth between channels without becoming overly emotional. He or she may simply observe, thinking, *Hmm, that's a good point . . . but the other side had a good point too!* However, mastering detachment is extremely hard, so the next best thing is to turn off the news.

You know, already, that practically everything in the news is negative. You know this, so why do you keep tuning into it? Too many of us are becoming emotionally and spiritually invested in the negative things that are going on around us. We see what's happening and jump on Twitter or Facebook to rant and rave. As I pointed out previously, those negative emotions are changing the physiology of your body at a cellular level.

Whether it's a conservative or liberal news outlet doesn't matter. Both sides are constantly spewing negativity, not positivity. They're on a low vibration, not a high vibration. In order to be healthy, you have to stay on as high a vibration as possible.

If you watch Fox or CNN or MSNBC, know that they're *trying* to get a reaction from you. They create fear, anger, and sadness, and those emotions are what goes into your body and causes disease—physical disease. Because you invite them every day into your lounge, you may feel you are buddies with Anderson or Bill, but these friends are harming your health. It's not only TV, but also, all the other news sources—online and in print.

Each media channel frames the world in a particular way, with a particular slant, in order to get you to tune into it. That is called *entertainment*. Modern TV news is nothing but entertainment. So my question is, are you entertained by the drama of the world?

The biggest objection I hear when I tell someone to do this is, "But how am I going to know what's going on?" Here is my answer: "How profoundly does it really matter that you know what's going on? If something really horrible is happening—let's say, a natural disaster—your neighbors will come and tell you. Someone will call you, especially if it's likely to affect you directly. Realize that if you turn off the TV or the radio, if you close the newspaper or the Internet browser on your laptop, you will be absolutely fine and still know

## Your Mind

what's going on. If you want to lower your level of stress, it's essential to get away from the media!

We are living in a time when this is more important than ever before. Politics has become inescapable. It has torn families and friendships apart. It's interesting; I've gone to several metaphysical, New-Age conferences—which are generally supposed to be about love, healing, and positivity. But even there, I've heard people spew negativity about others with whom they don't agree on politics. Now if you love everybody, and you realize that we're all connected, why are you so hateful? Does it stem from self-hatred? People who are full of hate need to turn around and look more closely at themselves.

### Method Six: Declutter

One of the important pieces of being truly well in body, mind, and spirit is to make sure that you always get rid of junk and toxic material. That includes people, places, and things. Too much junk makes us miserable. It's important to understand the necessity for doing it, to feel good about doing it, and also have some strategies that can really work to allow you to move forward in your life and be well when you get rid of all kinds of junk.

*Your Smartphone*

Every January 1, I start looking through my cell phone contacts, and I try to identify the people about whom I have negative feelings. Using my practice of spiritual self-evaluation,

I ask myself, "What is this negative feeling about? Did they hurt or upset me once too often?"

Sometimes, though, you may come across people whom *you're* not serving. This might include those whom you're wrongfully enabling or those whom you have treated poorly or neglected too often. You're not right for everybody!

Whenever I feel that a relationship is not worth repairing at the present time, I do it: I press delete. It can be hard, but if you feel a person should go, here's a process for healthy deletion:

- Forgive that person for whatever he or she did.
- Forgive yourself.
- Press delete.

You may think that sounds really radical, but deleting these people from your phone is not only a great way to free up some memory on your device; it is also a healthy exercise in "letting go." It is like freeing up space in your brain and creating the space in your life to let in more people.

That act of letting go can create an energy break and make a difference. That doesn't mean you can never contact the person again. You know there are other ways to get in touch with most people you know if you really need them. Also, if you make a "mistake" and you're meant to be in the relationship after all, they will come back to you in some type of positive way.

However, each year I find I'm deleting fewer and fewer people, because I've become more patient and tolerant. I realize that when people who are difficult come into my life, perhaps they're there to teach me something.

**Your Space**

I'm incredulous when I watch the TV show *Hoarders*, but I realize that, over time, a lot of people (myself included) continue to collect stuff, and we don't necessarily throw away anything. It builds up without us noticing, but it's good practice to just start throwing away as much as you can. Get rid of stuff and make space in your life. Make space in your house. Make space in your car. Make space in your closets for air and for health. Go through everything, including your cabinets and your food. Once a month, look in your refrigerator and ask yourself, "Do I need this? What can I do with this?" If you can't do anything with it, just dump it in the trash and vow to buy only groceries you need in the future.

Purge your closets too. Many of us have clothes that are many different sizes, because many of us have *been* different sizes. Go through everything. Is there something that you really, absolutely love? Then keep it. But for every item you keep, you have to give away one item. Every year, make it a practice to let things go. If you can let go of physical objects, you will find it easier to let go of emotional baggage.

But decluttering isn't simply about throwing away things; it's about getting rid of *junk*. Junk isn't just stuff that has no value;

# But Now I See

it is also stuff that is physically bad for us. We'll talk about junk food later, but there are other kinds of junk you should toss out.

Look around your house, look around your place of employment, and ask yourself, "Are there any substances or things in my environment that could be making me sick?" Think about how you cook your food. Are you using the microwave a lot? There are studies that show that using a microwave can cause changes in food, and even being around the device can cause problems in your body. Warm up everything on the stove or in a conventional oven. If you must use a microwave, warm up things in glass containers rather than plastic ones. Get rid of non-stick cookware that contains toxic chemicals and use other cookware.

Use laundry detergent that doesn't have dyes and perfumes in it. Take a look at your cosmetics and your soaps, everything you use on a daily basis, and decrease your toxic load. Look around your house. It may be that you have old carpeting, that you have mold, that you have all types of toxins around you that are making you sick. This is a way to get rid of junk. There are plenty of online resources that provide information on toxins and products to steer clear of, so do your research and then change your buying habits.

### Method Seven: Laugh!

Americans have become so very serious—so angry—and we don't laugh enough. Laughing heals. Laughing makes us feel good. Laughing changes the physiology of our body. Our

## Your Mind

fear, anger, and sadness manifest in our body, and they harm it, but our loves and joys promote health. Laughter is the ultimate expression of joy. Life is stranger than fiction, and it's funny. Laugh and heal yourself instead of getting angry.

### Method Eight: Meditation

The above list of ways to boost mental wellbeing could go on for several more pages! There are so many more ways to feel good inside: taking long walks in nature, painting or drawing, owning a pet, and volunteering for a local charity, etc. Do whatever works for you, but be sure to put mental wellbeing at the top of your list of priorities. If you do, you'll notice the difference in your body in many ways.

***There's a reason they call it "irritable" bowel syndrome.*** Irritable people get irritable bowel syndrome. If you're having a digestive issue, it may be time to evaluate if there is something in your personality that is magnifying what's going on in your digestive system. The fact that positive behavior therapy—a type of psychological and emotional treatment—can help people with irritable bowel syndrome have fewer symptoms demonstrates the link between what's going on in your mind and in your digestive system.

If you have frequent bouts of constipation, it could be that you're holding on to too much. Do you retain all of your emotions? Do you never forgive? Can you not forget? Do you ruminate on things that happened years and years ago?

Letting go of the "crap" and the anger in your life will help your body relax, and the constipation will ease. If you do not tend to what's going on in your emotions and your spirit, there is no way you will ever be able to heal your body. This is the best news of all, because it means that you have the power. You have the power to change your body!

**Staying sane in this crazy world of ours can be tough, but mental strength will enable you to make it through whatever challenges life throws at you. Never neglect your mind; it might save your life!**

## Gift 5: Single-Question Reading

You may have one deep, burning question to which you have always wanted to know the answer. Perhaps there is one thing that you know is affecting your life and you want to determine what you can do about it. My areas of greatest intuition are health matters and romantic matters, and I may be able to help you find the answer you're seeking. Visit the link below and ask that one question today!

drveronica.wufoo.com/forms/
special-offer-single-question-reading/

Chapter 6

# Your Body (Part I)

*"Your body is a vehicle of your emotions and a vehicle of feelings and a vehicle of whatever you need to get done in life. And you've got to take care of that vehicle."*
—Eva Longoria, American Actress

In the last chapter, I mentioned the importance of loving yourself—not the narcissistic kind of love that sucks all the oxygen out of room, but the kind of love that enables you to love yourself despite your imperfections.

Although you may be overweight, look in the mirror and into your eyes and say, "I love you. Then fake it till you make it. However, you need to stop deluding yourself and making excuses such as, "It's in my genes. Everyone in my family is fat!" No more excuses. By loving yourself and being truly committed to yourself, you can be fit and healthy despite being in a family that isn't either of these things. My tough-love statement about this is, "Stop making excuses for being less than God desires you to be."

Remember that no food tastes as good as being healthy feels! Find a way to begin enjoying healthy food. To truly love yourself, you need to treat yourself well by eating the right foods and taking care of your body. You're living within yourself every day, so treat that place with respect. You wouldn't leave toxic-smelling trash lying around your apartment, so don't bring it into your body either! If you aren't a fan of health food, don't feel defeated! I have seen many people begin to love healthy food simply because they have begun to love themselves. Once they gain some self-esteem, they stop craving the bad food and hunger for the good stuff instead. They can still eat the bad food (potato chips and gummy bears, in my case), but their taste buds literally change when they feel better about themselves, and they begin to choose food that makes them feel good.

In this chapter, I'm going to focus on how to get in physical shape: diet and exercise. But I won't be giving you recipes or regimes to follow because the food one can eat and the exercise one can perform is specific to every individual. Rather, the purpose of this chapter is to give you some things to consider before you search for the solutions that are right for you.

# Your Body (Part I)

## Same Old Story

Day after day, I have people who come to me, and to my seminars, and ask, "What's the answer?" Oftentimes, they expect the answer to be found in a pill. They have an illness or injuries that have been a problem for a long time, yet they continue to do the same thing over and over again: go to the doctor, get the pills, take the pills. And when the problem returns, the same process is repeated. If you're sick or injured, that's a sign from the universe that you have to *change* something.

If you have high blood pressure, you have to change something! If you have diabetes, you've got to change something! Even if you fall down and hurt yourself, you might have to change something; your falls may be due to the way you walk or a problem with balance. The people who are able to read these road signs are the people who move on in life.

However, sometimes change will not be enough. A problem in your body may be simply be part of your journey through this life, a part of your story, and there could be a reason that it's staying with you. You shouldn't take that to mean you should just sit back and accept it, saying, "Oh, well. Being three hundred pounds is just a cross I must bear in this life." You must try. Don't become stuck repeating the same cycle of doctor appointments and prescriptions. Doing the same thing over and over and expecting different results is thought by some to be the definition of insanity. Get off the insanity train!

## The Wellness Pie

There are five equal-sized parts to the wellness pie:

- Nutrition
- Fitness
- Nervous System
- Hormones
- Detoxification

Each piece counts for 20 percent, so the good news is that, even if all you do is eat well, you can enjoy improvement in your health and wellness. To achieve *complete* wellness, however, you must attend to the other 80 percent as well. We've touched on some of these pieces already, and some we'll get to later. But for now, I want to focus on fitness.

## Exercise

Fitness is 20 percent of the whole picture, but you must have that 20 percent to get to 100 percent. The other 80 percent has to be tended to in order for you to achieve vitality and longevity. I stress that it's 20 percent because most people's wellness plan includes just two things: diet and exercise, which are given fifty-fifty status.

When it comes to your fitness, twenty is the magic number. In addition to being the percentage of the wellness pie, twenty is the number of minutes you need to exercise and the number of days per month you need to exercise. For those who really

## Your Body (Part I)

hate to move, this is more good news! You can complete your entire exercise routine in only twenty minutes.

Science proves that, for just about everybody, high-intensity interval training is effective. A twenty-minute routine four times a week will produce lasting results. High-intensity interval training is beautiful because it is performed in short bursts, alternating between resting, exercising moderately, and exercising intensely for twenty minutes. Why is this important? It's been shown that it boosts your cardiovascular system in addition to building muscle. You want muscle because it burns more calories than fat does, and it burns them twenty-four hours a day. So the more muscle you have, the more calories you'll burn, keeping you fit even when you're not exercising. Find yourself a twenty-minute routine, perform it four times a week, and then you can call it a day.

It takes about a month of doing something regularly to turn it into a habit. Twenty of those thirty days should be when you exercise, while ten are your rest days. Rest days are important for your muscles.

### Whatever You Do, Do Something.

In addition to promoting weight loss, exercise is good for every single health condition. There are multiple research studies that show that every chronic illness—even serious ones—is improved by some type of fitness routine. For instance, there have been studies that show that women who have breast cancer are less likely to have a recurrence of the disease if they partake in exercise. Studies have also shown that people with arthritis feel less pain as a result of exercise—not more, as you might expect. We even know that people who have serious heart ailments and lung disease see improvements in their health through exercise. What kind of exercise you should perform is always up for debate, but the bottom line is, you should definitely get moving!

To be a bodybuilder or an elite athlete requires a certain amount of time and training. But for the average person to exercise, he or she just to move something, sometime. Realize that instead of sitting on your couch and watching TV, it is a better idea to take your dog on a longer walk than usual—even if it's only for ten minutes! Ten minutes is ten times more beneficial than moving for no minutes! Any amount of exercise is better than none at all, even if you have cancer, heart disease, lung disease, or any other type of serious illness that makes you feel like you don't want to move. The more you feel like you don't want to move, the more you probably *should* move.

It's worth reminding you that exercise is also beneficial to your mental health. I don't run as much as I used to, but I've always enjoyed the "runner's high." There would be a point in running when my mind would clear, and all of a sudden, I would get brilliant revelations and ideas.

# Your Body (Part I)

## Scales Can Lie

Please be mindful that there is such a thing as overtraining, which can increase the level of stress on your body. Once you're in the habit of fitness training, it can be highly addictive, and it's tempting for people to exercise more, assuming it will help them lose weight. But the scales can lie to us. We know this because we all know some skinny fat people.

For example, I have a good friend who is large woman, but in a medical evaluation, her numbers are some of the best numbers that you could possibly see. She has no health issues. It's important to point out that we all want our reflection to look a certain way. Even my friend, who has these great numbers, has a lot of angst because she looks a particular way in the mirror. There are other people who look just beautiful according to our societal standards, but they have horrible numbers that suggest that they are on the road to diabetes, cancer, heart disease, autoimmune disease, thyroid disease, and other ailments. Go for the numbers of wellness, which are those underlying numbers, not just what you see on the scale.

Why is the scale not telling you the whole story? Muscle weighs more than fat. When you do the right types of exercise and eat the right types of food, your body composition begins to change. You may look better in the mirror and your clothes fit better, but the number on the scale may not necessarily decrease. Don't feel defeated. Your goals should be physical wellness (energy, vitality, and longevity), not keeping the scale at a certain number.

To avoid the harm you can cause your body by training too hard, you should go slow to begin with and build up over time. You want to make sure that you only put a little bit of stress on your body—because that's been shown to be beneficial—and teach your body how to balance and adapt.

## Get Help from a Specialist: One Size Never Fits All

Don't just pick up the latest fad-diet book! It's not that easy.

At this point in time, there are about seven billion people on the planet. That means there are seven billion different ways of doing something. When you read about a new diet or exercise program online and decide that you're going to implement it, realize that there's a very slim chance that it's right for you! The important part of becoming fit is to learn something that you can do, that you enjoy, and that you can sustain for an extended period of time in your life.

I always recommend that people seek out a practitioner who understands more than, "Just lose weight and just do exercise." The practitioner has to understand where you are in your life and how to prescribe a particular type of exercise for you. You want a practitioner who knows the science of how different types of bodies work, and how different types of conditions develop, so that then he or she can use that science to give you a proper exercise and movement prescription. Once your practitioner helps you understand the science, you'll be able to figure out what the most beneficial form of movement is for you, as well as the best eating strategy.

I recommend that people have genetic sequencing through 23andme.com (see the end of this chapter for a $50 discount gift!). Once you know your genetic sequence, there are practitioners who know how to use this information to script your health plan. Simply learning what eating strategy, fitness plan, and supplements to use based on genetics can lead to remarkable improvements in a person's health.

But science is just one part. The complementary part is the inner you. You're in the state you're in because of your life's journey. A holistic and functional wellness practitioner can put your story on a timeline and into a matrix in order to figure out what the antecedents, triggers, and mediating factors were that have led you where you are today. Together, conventional and functional medicine practices can recommend a holistic program that will effectively help you on your path to healing.

## Your Body and Blood Type

What many fad diets and nutritionists fail to recognize is that when it comes to eating well and exercising right, one size does not fit all. Knowing what type of body you have, as well as the type blood that flows around it, can help you look after yourself more effectively. First, let's consider the body.

From a purely physiological standpoint, Western medicine simplifies our bodies by placing them into three categories:

**Endomorph:** People with this body type tend to store fat easily. Often these people are large all over, but sometimes they are pear shaped (storing fat in the hips and thighs) or apple shaped (storing fat mainly around the middle).

**Ecotomorph:** People who tend to be beanpole-thin and have difficulty building up their muscles.

**Mesomorph:** People who are mesomorphs are the lucky ones! They tend to be well built, have a high metabolism, and possess muscle cells that are responsive to workouts.

But Ayurvedic medicine goes further than the physio; it goes psycho! It's beyond the scope of this book to go into this in detail. It's your homework to go do some research—but here's a quick overview.

In the Indian Ayurvedic system, there are three psycho-physiological types known as "doshas" with names that make them sound more like sororities: Vata, Pitta, and Kapha. We are all predominantly one type, but it's more complicated than that because the doshas are dynamic energies that respond to a whole bunch of things, including how we feel, what we eat, and even the seasons. Each dosha relates to specific elements within our bodies (stomach, bones, joints, skin, etc.) and also to specific emotions (jealousy, joy, anger, etc.). The aim is to

## Your Body (Part I)

balance the doshas to enhance their positive attributes, not the negative ones. The doshas can be properly balanced with a tailored program of diet, exercise, and meditation.

A practitioner of functional medicine would advise figuring out where your doshas are balanced and imbalanced before you decide on any diet or exercise regime. There's no point in starving or tiring yourself for nothing!

Alternatively, in Traditional Chinese Medicine (TCM), there are five elements: wood, fire, earth, metal, and water. According to TCM, we all predominantly fit into one or two of these elements, and our bodies work differently according to which element we most embody. To help you gain a really great understanding of these elements and how they affect your health, I recommend the book *Let Magic Happen: Adventures in Healing with a Holistic Radiologist* by Dr. Larry Burk.

In addition to your body type, your blood type is also important. I'm most impressed by the work of Dr. Peter J. D'Adamo—one of the authors of *Eat Right 4 Your Type*—who shows that different types of exercise are beneficial to different people based on their blood type, which has to do with their genetic background. Some people are well suited for long-distance running, while other people are more suited for weightlifting. Still other people may be perfectly suited for Tai Chi. The idea is to find the exercise that is physiologically going to do the most for you, and realize that the answer is going to be different for everybody based on his or her ancestry.

Realize that you can read all the research and follow it, but you still may be doing the incorrect exercise for *you*. You have to find the exercise that works best for your blood type and your body type, and that exercise should be one that you're able to sustain.

## Diet: What You Eat Is Eating You

Whatever body and blood type you are, there are foods that are bad for *everyone*.

Diet is nobody's favorite subject, and I can almost hear you groaning from here! But when we talk about eating "clean" as you possibly can and following a whole-foods diet, it doesn't mean you can never eat fun food. All it means is that, for the most part, you're doing the best you can to eat clean.

We all know that we need food to survive, but how much food and what kind is still hotly disputed. There's a lot of debate in America about what is good food and what is not. There's even more debate about which diet plan you should be on. By the way, I don't like the word "diet" because it has "die" in the front; for me, it's a negative word. I prefer the term "eating strategies." We want to live, so how do we eat to live? How do we figure out what is the right strategy for each of us? Eating should always be enjoyable. It's about your soul and your spirit.

# Your Body (Part I)

Think about what food is and what it represents. The reason why people *love* certain foods so much is because they usually have a context in which they are eaten. It may be a family event or it may be associated with friends and fellowship. Food is not just about surviving; it is also about thriving, because the food you eat matters from a spiritual perspective. This is why dinners surrounding holidays are so fraught with emotion. There's so much discussion around where dinners are going to be, what will be on the menu, who will eat this but not that, etc. Our particular tastes might even have come to us from our mothers in the womb!

Because food matters to your body and your spirit, you always want your food to be prepared and consumed with love. Since food nourishes our body, our mind, and our soul, we have to pay attention to everything that we put in our mouth, and formulate a particular eating strategy to *live*.

So, until you are able to determine what body and blood type you are, what can you do to eat better?

## Food for Thought

Although I cannot offer you a specific diet plan here, I am going to highlight some general principles you should consider as you develop a new approach to healthy eating.

## Stay Away from Whitey

White foods are almost always bad for us. If it's white, it's probably been refined, and highly refined foods in our diet are inflammatory. In practically everybody I have done energetic testing on, I find some type of reaction to refined food. White foods break up the energetic field; people have negative response to them, which means they are throwing their body out of balance. What tends to make white foods even worse in the American culture is that these foods tend to be genetically modified and overprocessed.

I found out that I'm allergic to certain American-made foods, and one of those foods is wheat. Not all gluten—but wheat, specifically. It interrupts my energy field. When I eat too much of it, I notice certain parts of my body will get inflamed. I have a knee injury, and if I eat too much white flour (like a lot of bread) my knee will start hurting. I also had a little injury in my elbow, and too much wheat can make it hurt. Other times, wheat can cause me to become bloated.

However, when I travel out of the country, in places where the food is less processed, not genetically modified, and not covered in as many pesticides, I tend not to have a lot of reactions. For instance, on my trip to France, I ate bread every single day, *every single day*, and suffered no bloating and no inflammation in my knee. I cannot do that in America unless I can find organic sources of wheat. Even then, I still have a reaction and it does still interrupt my energetic field. However, there are other factors that come into play here in America that stop me from being able to eat wheat—organic or processed—safely.

# Your Body (Part I)

We all like a little bit of sweetness; some people like it more than others. But we don't have to rely on white, refined sugar; there are different ways to experience sweetness. One natural source is Stevia, which is herbal. You can also get raw, organic sugar, which tends to be brown and more flavorful. Honey is a great, natural source of sweetness, as well, and it's good for you in other ways. Always look for an alternative to white sugar.

What else? Rice. I ask people in my seminars, "What rice is better? White rice or brown rice?" Everybody answers "brown." White rice is known to be more refined, so people assume brown is better. However, there's a caveat to it. In the Ayurvedic system, my dominant dosha is Pitta, and guess what? Pittas do better with white rice than brown rice! Now I understand why I experience stomach upset when I have more brown rice, but when I eat white rice, I'm fine. So, perhaps white *can* be right!

Let's talk about potatoes. Regular types of white potato tend to be worse for the body than their darker skinned companions, including sweet potatoes and red potatoes, which tend to contain more nutrients. So, if you want the healthy potatoes, think about eating the rainbow, as opposed to the white ones.

Can you have some white potatoes? Yes. Can you have some white rice? Yes. Can you have some white sugar? Yes. Can you have wheat? Yes. But if you eat it all in balanced and limited quantities, you're going to be a lot better off because these four foods cause a lot of inflammation. If you want to do *one thing* for your health, just stay away from white.

### Feeling Blue

It's a little-known fact that, to select a proper eating strategy, each of us should take into account where we are from. This theory is laid out in Dan Buettner's wonderful book, *The Blue Zones*, which identifies the geographic areas of the world where the people live the longest and the healthiest. These places are called "Blue Zones."

There are five blue zones: Ogliastra Region, Sardinia; Okinawa, Japan; Loma Linda, California; Nicoya Peninsula, Costa Rica; and Ikaria, Greece. People who live in these very different parts of the world have low rates of disease and tend to live longer than the average population in other parts of the world. Of course, other non-food factors contribute to their longevity—exercise, level of happiness, community service, and so on—but the most significant factor is nutrition.

Despite differences in genetics and the diets across the zones, all the people have one thing in common: they're not eating processed foods—unlike most Americans. Processed foods form the bulk of an average American's diet because it's cheap and convenient, but it's killing us.

The author of *The Blue Zones* tells us that the Blue Zone populations' healthy eating is supplemented by health-promoting factors that we can all incorporate into our lives:

# Your Body (Part I)

1. Move naturally (have an active life).
2. Cut calories by 20 percent.
3. Avoid processed foods.
4. Drink red wine (in moderation).
5. Take time to see the big picture.
6. Take time to relieve stress.
7. Participate in a spiritual community.
8. Make family a priority.
9. Be surrounded by those who share Blue Zone values.

## Refine Your Palette (and Your Palate)

Think of your plate as an artist's palette and aim for as much variety of color as you can. You want all different colors in your diet because they represent different nutrients that your body needs. Taking vitamin supplements may not be as effective as consuming them in natural foods, so eat as many colors as you possibly can! It is best to get your vitamins through your food—especially fresh, whole foods.

### Red

- Tomatoes, pomegranates, beets, radishes, red berries
- Leads to healthy bones, decreases inflammation, creates better immunity, good for healthy eyes/skin/hair

### Green

- Leafy greens, broccoli, cucumber, asparagus, avocado
- Good for eyes, lungs, and liver, lowers blood pressure, aids cell production

### Yellow/Orange

- Bananas, carrots, pumpkin, citrus fruits, sweet potato, pineapple
- Reduces risk of heart disease and cancer, leads to increased immunity, decreases inflammation

### Blue/Purple

- Red onions, eggplant, blueberries, purple cabbage
- Protects cells from damage, improve memory, longer life

### Neutral

- Onions, cauliflower, garlic, parsnips, mushrooms
- Lowers cholesterol, increases immunity, good for skin/hair/eyes

### Everything in Moderation

When I went to France, I got a little sniffle. My brother-in-law offered me cognac. After I shot back a couple glasses of cognac, I wasn't drunk, but my sniffles went away instantly. A little cognac, a little Bordeaux, a little bit of this, a little bit of that; this is how the French do it. I always learn a lot when I go to France to visit with my husband's family. You might be saying, "But I've never been to France, so how do I know what to do?" Well, rather than go into it here, I recommend a book by Mireille Guiliano: *French Women Don't Get Fat: The Secret of* Eating for Pleasure.

## Your Body (Part I)

It's fine to have variety in your diet, but don't overdo it! You can eat great food and enjoy a lot of pleasure doing so. Sit down, as the French do, to enjoy your company and the scenery along with the food. If at all possible, try taking a two-hour lunch once a week. If you have an understanding boss, tell him or her that you will be much more productive in the afternoon because you will have had time to unwind, digest food, and dream up new ideas.

### Shop the Perimeter

When you go shopping, stay around the edges of the store. All the foods you need to stay healthy can be found along the perimeter of the store. This is where you can find fresh meat and fish, fruit, vegetables, eggs, and dairy products. Once you step into the aisles, you're in trouble, because the shelves are stacked with processed foods. If you do venture into the world of bottles, cans, and packets, make sure that you read the ingredients list. Aim to only buy foods that contain no more than six ingredients, and you should know what those ingredients actually *are*.

Eating should be joyful and fun! The processed stuff might be delicious, but there is no fun in eating something that will make you sick. True joy comes from eating well-made, clean food that will make your body strong and fit.

## Look after Your Digestion

In the last chapter, I raised the issue of irritable bowel syndrome as a problem related to your emotions. However, clearly your digestive system can fall victim to poor diet.

Our digestive system is the most important system in our body. It's where we get all our nutrients, and it's where we release our toxins, but you may be surprised to learn that 70 percent of the immune system is in the digestive system. When people get sick, it is likely that their digestive system is broken.

You've got to clean and repair from top to bottom because the digestive system is like a river that flows downhill. If there is something wrong in your mouth, it can affect what's going wrong the rest of the way down. If there's something wrong in your stomach, it can affect what is going on in your colon or your small intestine. If something is wrong in your small intestine, it can affect what's going on in your large intestine.

So how should you go about cleaning up your digestive system? It's certainly not about getting a colonoscopy or an endoscopy. It's about eating the right foods and getting the right nutrients into your digestive system.

One of the pillars of maintaining health is detoxification. A few times a year, it's recommended that you detox. There are several different detox methods. Colonics can be helpful for some people, but most people can achieve good results with

## Your Body (Part I)

eating strategies, plus supplements, and drainage support to be able to clean out their body a couple of times a year.

I don't recommend a water or juice fast. There was a study out of Taiwan that showed that people actually become *more* toxic when they do a juice cleanse or a water cleanse. A healthcare practitioner should be consulted to put together a detoxification program that's suited to your particular body, including your underlying medical condition.

**The key to successful weight loss is an eating strategy that is right for your body type. Take the time to understand how your body works inside and out, and you'll soon see the difference.**

### Gift 6: Your Health Score

I know you are looking for a way to determine where you're at in terms of overall health. Fill out this questionnaire, and see where you come out. This questionnaire yields a score that you can use over time to track your health progress.

How healthy are you? drveronica.wufoo.com/forms/how-healthy-are-you/

### Gift 7: 23andme.com Discount

Use this link to get a $50 discount: 23andme.com/drveronica

Chapter 7

# Your Body (Part II)

In the last chapter, we focused on poor diet and lack of exercise as key reasons for unhealthiness, but there's more going on. In this chapter, therefore, we will turn to the physical effects of stress because no amount of healthy eating or the right kind of exercise will help you if hormonal or chemical imbalances are holding you back.

## Signaling to the Universe

There are numerous laws that govern how the universe works, and without realizing, you are sending out signals into space, like NASA sends out signals to the space station. We are constantly interacting with the universe, but most people do so based on the way they *believe* that everything works. This mostly involves "traditional" science: biology and chemistry.

But there's also quantum physics, which is the science of energy on the atomic and subatomic levels. Quantum physics determines the way our own energy systems interact, and the people who've figured out how to change their energy rapidly, in the blink of an eye, have miraculous healings.

To master your body, to master your spirit, you have to practice transforming your energy. The Creator has put in place the laws of the universe. Once you learn them, practice them, and master them, you can meditate and bring about energy transformations.

There are twelve laws in the universe that aren't taught to us by religion or in school, but they are laws that we are all subject to. People who understand these laws will be able to better understand how to get their life to go the way they want it to go, and that includes their health. But before we get into the twelve laws, let me just say that this isn't just woo-woo stuff; these are a combination of spiritual, physical, and scientific laws that visionaries such as Albert Einstein, Napoleon Hill, and Deepak Chopra have all investigated and written about.

**The Law of Divine Oneness:** Everything is connected through God because God is omnipresent. We are all part of God's energy. And because we are all connected, whatever we do (or think) affects everyone and everything else.

**Law of Vibration:** All particles travel in circular patterns and our thoughts, feelings, and desires behave the same way.

## Your Body (Part II)

**Law of Action:** To make things happen, we must do things that make them happen. Our actions should correspond to our thoughts, dreams, emotions, and words.

**Law of Correspondence:** All the laws of physics at the universal level apply at the human level on Earth.

**Law of Cause and Effect:** Nothing happens by chance. Every action (including thought) has a reaction.

**Law of Compensation:** Our good deeds are rewarded.

**Law of Attraction:** Everything we do has an energy that attracts similar energies. Negative attracts negatives; positive attract positives.

**The Law of Perpetual Transmutation of Energy:** Everyone has the power to change the conditions of their lives through the exchange of low energy for high energy.

**Law of Relativity:** Challenges present themselves to us for a reason (opportunities to learn and grow and strengthen our inner light), and all problems are relative to the problems of others who might be worse off.

**Law of Polarity:** Everything bad has a polar opposite of good. By focusing on the good pole, we can overcome the bad.

**Law of Rhythm:** Everything moves and vibrates to certain rhythms, e.g., seasons, life cycles, etc. We need to stay in flow throughout these rhythms of life.

**Law of Gender:** Everything and everyone has feminine and masculine sides and energies; this is how creation occurs in the universe. We must all find the balance between the two to master our lives.

To discuss each of these laws in detail is beyond the scope of this book. But there is plenty of information out there for you to read if you're interested in knowing more. For now, simply understand that, like the laws of the road (what a stop sign or the red, yellow, and green lights mean), the laws of the universe will guide you to the correct path in certain life situations.

Your own energy system is interacting with everything that's going on in the universe. You are able to make changes by choice. There is no "out there" that's controlling you like a marionette. *You* decide how you're going to do things. People who are ignorant of these laws engage in behaviors that are counterproductive to their life. The people who are masters of these laws are those who have the best life, the best health, the best house. They have the best of everything because they have mastered the laws of the universe.

But how do you master the laws? You can't simply read how-to books; you need to learn by doing and being taught by someone who has already become a master. These individuals—masters and teachers—are outside of your box; you are trapped inside of the box and cannot see clearly. They can see and show you where you're going wrong. It's akin to

## Your Body (Part II)

learning how to drive and having somebody in the car to tell you exactly what to do and correct your errors. As your driving improves, you'll need the instructor less and less until, finally, you can drive alone.

There are lots of books, courses, and retreats that can help people change their energy and learn different healing principles. To plant the seed of curiosity in your mind, go on an exploration of what is possible. I recommend that you start by searching for and watching an incredible YouTube video entitled "Gregg Braden, Bladder Cancer Dissolves in Less Than 3 Minutes Using the Language of Emotion." In it, Gregg says, "It's only a miracle until we understand the science." This video will inspire you to continue your education in what is possible.

Now it's time look at what the signals you're sending out might be.

### Chemical Signals

Your body's chemicals—its neurotransmitters—have to be in balance for life to be OK physically, spiritually, and emotionally. But what are these chemicals?

**Serotonin** is one of the "happy" chemicals that many of you will have heard of. It is widely considered to be responsible for mood balance, and if it's in short supply, depression may result. Although it's thought of as a brain chemical, it's mostly found in the gastrointestinal tract, and, therefore, it is important to your digestion too. Serotonin levels are also thought to affect sexual appetite, memory, sleep patterns, and bone density, among many other things. You can influence the levels of serotonin naturally through exercise and diet, but also via light therapy.

**Dopamine** is a neurotransmitter that helps control the brain's pleasure centers. It is also sometimes called the "motivational molecule" because it is related to concentration and productivity. Low levels of dopamine can cause mood swings, poor sex drive, memory loss, and more. You can increase your dopamine levels by eating a diet rich in tyrosine, an amino acid found in foods such as chocolate (woo-hoo!), coffee (again, woo-hoo!), almonds, and oatmeal.

**Norepinephrine** functions as both a hormone and a neurotransmitter, and its role is to spur the body and brain into action. It is associated with mental disorders, such as ADHD. On the plus side, it helps us focus and remember things, but on the other hand, it can also contribute to anxiety and depression. The chemical's other functions include increasing blood pressure and triggering the release of energy in the form of glucose. Foods containing tyrosine help to naturally boost norepinephrine.

When the chemicals in the brain are working as they should be, we're happy, we're in balance, we want to eat right, we are nice to people, and we're nice to ourselves. But when a chemical gets out of balance, we want the salt, the candy, the

## Your Body (Part II)

cigarette; we want to gamble and to have sex for the sake of sex. We want to do all the things that are counterproductive to our general wellbeing. An imbalance of these chemicals also leads to issues like irritable bowel syndrome, pain, chronic fatigue, and weight gain.

I often meet overweight and depressed people. But which came first, the fatness or the sadness? Those who are overweight are more likely to have out-of-balance brain chemicals—number one being serotonin—and people are being medicated with antidepressants. But a good diet and exercise program can naturally raise serotonin levels! It is possible to medicate women who suffer from a low sex drive with a dopamine pill, but again, with diet and exercise, libido can be raised naturally.

### Hormonal Signals

Hormones, along with the neurotransmitting chemicals, regulate everything that goes on in our body. There are hundreds of types of hormones in the body, but there are a few that can cause major problems when they are out of balance.

Here are just a few of the hormones that are very important in weight control:

**Leptin:** This hormone signals to your brain that you're full and don't need that dessert, thankyouverymuch. Fat produces leptin, so if you have a lot of fat, your brain becomes resistant to the signals leptin sends.

**Estrogen:** This hormone in high levels can make you insulin-resistant, resulting in the storage of glucose as fat in your body. A diet lacking in fiber can drive up estrogen levels. A decrease in estrogen can raise the level of leptin (see above), so it's important to keep the balance just right.

**Testosterone:** This hormone (present in women too) is needed for a healthy metabolism. Too little of it, and we can't burn calories effectively and they're turned into to fat.

**Thyroid:** The thyroid basically sends out signals to the rest of the body about how fast or slowly you should use and burn your energy. If your thyroid is slow, you're going to gain weight.

**Cortisol:** This is our stress hormone, or the "fight or flight" hormone. When we're under stress, it helps us to get away from danger; it allows us to react to circumstances and preserve our life. But these days, people feel constantly stressed. When its level is out of balance, cortisol can cause weight gain because what do we do when we're stressed? We eat and drink too much!

Not only can your hormones make you fat, they can also make you sick. If your cortisol is out of balance, it can affect your immune system too. This is why, when you're stressed, you tend to be more susceptible to illnesses like the common cold. Also understand that cortisol levels have been implicated in conditions like chronic fatigue syndrome and fibromyalgia, and too much estrogen is implicated in insulin resistance and diabetes, as well as polycystic ovarian syndrome.

# Your Body (Part II)

There are ways to balance many of these hormones by utilizing certain eating strategies, vitamin supplements, herbal remedies, and other therapeutic practices. Don't just resort to a prescription! When you balance your hormones—and you *can* balance them—you will feel good and be energetic.

## Killer Stress

But what causes hormonal imbalance? My answer to that may seem flippant: "anything and everything." But, honestly, the number-one cause of hormonal imbalance is stress. If you have had all the tests, you're eating the right foods, and you're doing the right types of exercise, but your body is still not working right, you must evaluate what is going on in your life, your mind, your spirit, and your past lives.

I consult with so many people who have health problems and whose lives are falling apart in some way. Their ill health is their hormones saying, "I can't take this anymore. I'm gonna make your hair fall out, make your blood pressure too high, make you have a stroke, give you irritable bowel syndrome, make you walk crookedly, give you Hashimoto's disease, give you cancer . . ." But as soon as the person realizes it's their hormones, the body begins to respond positively, as if to say, "Thank you for finally listening to me and doing something about that awful husband, that crappy job situation, that pity party, that lack of self-love . . ."

Moving to a new place, having a baby, getting married, losing a parent, being sick, crashing the car, worrying about job security. Our lives are full of highly stressful situations. But stress can be more low-key, and sometimes it's hard to pinpoint what we are stressed about. People might think, *Why do I just feel so discontented?* Perhaps they look at their lives and see no reason to feel discontented, yet that nagging feeling of dissatisfaction persists.

The big picture is that people have to understand that life is always going to have its challenges. That's what life is about; it's one challenge, then the next, then the next. This is how we all grow and evolve.

A problem arises when people become chronically stressed. I was having a discussion with a friend over lunch recently who complained, "I'm just always so angry! I've always been angry. I don't really know why. Maybe it's because my mother was angry?" He had begun to dig deep and evaluate why he is so angry, which is a good start. Stressed-out parents can certainly raise stressed-out children. You have to realize that all your stress and energy is sending out signals to the universe from a spiritual state that is not conducive to bringing children into the world. Stress, anger, and unhappiness are often learned behaviors rather than the result of actual, real-life problems. Sometimes there are physical reasons that people behave in certain ways—imbalances that can explain why a person is stressed or depressed.

## Your Body (Part II)

We can stay locked within those health-harming emotions or we can figure out how to escape by asking what we are supposed to learn from this stressful situation. In being more dispassionate, you can transform your emotions into the health-promoting kind. Being able to move on from negative events is critical to your health, but it does not mean that you're going to be able to switch off the full spectrum of emotions; you can't be 100 percent happy all of the time. You do have the ability to recognize stress and the emotions that don't seem so productive, and read the signs that it's time to do something more positive.

You have to realize that your energy is sending out signals to the universe from a spiritual state. If your spirit is in a state of constant stress, it will lead to stress in your body, and nowhere is the invisible stress of your spirit and your life more evident than in your reproductive system.

### Stress and Fertility

When we're in a state of self-protection—the state we enter when we're highly stressed—the last thing we're thinking about is reproducing. It's meant to be like that; it's an instinct. When we are running from a lion, we're certainly not thinking about sex! Today, we're not running from carnivorous cats, but we're running from our boss, our finances, and our relationships, and guess what? Fertility problems in men and women are on the rise.

Stress raises the level of the cortisol hormone. The cortisol helps you deal with the stress, but it means that the sex hormones—testosterone and estrogen—cannot compete. In brief, the science behind this is that cholesterol (it is a good substance too!) is needed before the production of cortisol, progesterone, estrogen, and testosterone is made possible. When you're under stress, more of the cholesterol is going toward the production of cortisol, and less toward the other hormones that promote fertility.

This is something that's often overlooked in people who are dealing with fertility problems. Yes, there are physical problems that can be addressed, but stress is a big factor. And, of course, if you're trying to get pregnant but cannot, that itself will raise your stress levels, making it even harder to conceive. We've all heard about the person who was trying and trying to get pregnant but gave up in frustration only to fall pregnant soon afterward. She let go of the frustration and the stress, and lo and behold, a year later, she has a baby.

It's hard to determine which came first in this chicken-or-egg situation—the stress or the infertility. You may never discover the answer to that question. However, you can be sure that the reason for infertility is not God punishing you. Realize that if you're having issues with fertility, it's time not just for a physical evaluation, but also a spiritual and emotional evaluation. There's a reason for everything. What is your spiritual or emotional problem that's leading to your infertility?

First, ask yourself if there is a spiritual blockage of any kind, something that is giving you doubts or causing you stress.

## Your Body (Part II)

Total honesty is essential because you're asking yourself some tough questions, such as: "Am I really ready for a child?" or, "Is my partner truly excited have children?" "Are there still issues about my own childhood that I need to resolve before I can have a child of my own?" or, "Do I want a baby for the right reasons?" "Am I confident I can be a good father?" You have to evaluate what's going on in your spirit that could be leading to your difficulties in producing a child of your own.

In dealing with infertility, traditional and complementary medicine can work wonders where physical issues exist. Fertility doctors have a vast range of tests at their disposal to examine the underlying physical cause, and they can prescribe certain drugs to optimize the chances of conception. But conventional medicine may not have the complete answer. What many healthcare providers fail to tell their patients is that the ways to fix fertility issues include natural, holistic therapies, such as acupuncture and hypnosis, which can be quite effective. The whole universe is made up of energy, and everything we see around us is made up of energy. Complementary-medicine practitioners can help patients change their energy system. For instance, if you are stressed about family, you may be likely to have problems located in your root or baseline energy system. A disturbance in the root or baseline energy system can contribute to bone or blood diseases, or problems in your lower limbs. Complementary medicines, such as Ayurveda and TCM, have a clear and well-defined method of dealing with energy systems in manner that traditional medicine cannot.

### Many Are Called but Few Are Chosen

Understandably, infertility is a touchy subject. And the fact is that there are plenty of physically and spiritually fit people who, sadly, simply cannot reproduce.

I am a birth mother, as well as an adoptive mother, so I can appreciate firsthand that sometimes a woman who has chosen to birth children is not always also chosen to be a mother, and one who is unable to birth her own children may still be called to be a mother, a mother to many. In other words, motherhood and fatherhood are not necessarily biological terms. Often, being maternal or paternal is a way of being, a state of mind, a calling.

Understand that part of your spiritual story—and part of what is going on in your life—may be that you are chosen to parent in a way other than giving birth. What you have to ask yourself is, "What or who am I going to mother?" It may be that the reason you have not been chosen in this life to birth a child is because you have another purpose, and that purpose would be deterred if you had your own birth child. Practically every woman believes she's called to motherhood, but the question is *how* are you chosen? Have you created the right environment to be chosen to give birth? Or, on a spiritual level, have you been chosen by other souls to be their mother?

## Your Body (Part II)

You can be chosen to be a birth mother and have a baby, but you can also be chosen to be an adoptive mother who takes care of a baby and raises him or her to adulthood.

I know the pleasure of being both a birth mother and an adoptive mother, and both are wonderful. I am blessed that I've been chosen, not just by my birth sons, but also by my adoptive son. Realize that you may be chosen by a child, by a soul, by a being whom you will not birth, but who wants you to be his or her mother or father.

Remember when earlier we explored vibrations we looked at gratitude, love, and joy as being highest on the vibration spectrum. Keeping these emotions at the forefront of your life, even through the challenges, will help you in your quest to find out what kind of parent you're called to be, or if that is even your calling at all. You can eat all the right foods, take all the right supplements, but if you have not mastered gratitude, love, and joy, you will be too stressed to find true fulfillment and health.

**If Satan did indeed exist, he would not physically appear on Earth as a red guy with a pitchfork; rather, he would manifest himself more stealthily in the form of stress! Stress has the power to utterly destroy us in body, mind, and spirit, so do your best to banish it from your life. Never let stress in and never let it win.**

## Gift 8: Living Matrix Health Assessment

Having your entire history laid out on a timeline, including all the factors and events that have affected your health, can be transformative in guiding you and wise practitioners to the results you desire for your health. The Matrix points to one of seven areas that can be problematic. Check out this sample report: drveronica.com/living-matrix-evaluation/

And then get your Living Matrix Health Assessment:

drveronica.wufoo.com/forms/
special-offer-living-matrix-evaluation-297/

# Reflections

Well, we have arrived at the end of the book, and it's nearly time for us to part ways. We've covered a lot of ground, from the mysteries of woo-woo to the respective dangers of both doctrine and doctoring, from the importance of physical health to the threats facing your mental health, and from spiritual evaluation to stress limitation. Of course, there are many more things I would like to talk to you about, but I don't want to overwhelm you with too many big ideas all at once. So, it is with some reluctance that I now bid you a fond farewell.

Before I go, I would like to leave you with a message of hope and power. After reading this book, you should have hope that you have the insight into what your spirit is telling you about your health. Your power comes from your new knowledge that you are able to change what's going on in your spirit and emotion, and thereby have an impact on what's going on in your body.

I hope you are now convinced that your body, mind, and soul are all interconnected. The universe has made your life this way; the Creator of all has made it this way. Armed with this information, you understand that the ability to bring about a miracle healing lies within you; the power is in reach.

Having come to the end of this book, take a few days to meditate on its contents, using the new habit of spiritual self-evaluation we explored in Chapter 4. What concepts within this book spoke to you? What ideas are you still doubtful about? What was revealed to you about your own life and how you're living it? You may find that what you learned in this book only begins to resonate in the days and weeks to come. That's how it should be. The lesson you learn in life may not be clear at the time, but the more you reflect, the stronger your understanding of the lesson's importance will become. The purpose of your life is to understand what you are taught, and deep learning should never be rushed. The secret of life is to always "stay in school" and never stop learning because to learn is to grow, and we all know what it means when something stops growing: it begins to die.

However, do not make the mistake of believing that this book is the end of your journey of self-discovery. This book is only the beginning. It is intended to inspire you to go out

## Reflections

and explore your spirituality and learn how spiritual matters affect your bodily health.

If you're not sure where to turn next, here is my list of my favorite resources that I've mentioned throughout this book, which you, too, might find illuminating:

- *Many Lives, Many Masters: The True Story of a Prominent Psychiatrist, His Young Patient, and the Past-Life Therapy That Changed Both Their Lives* by Brian L. Weiss, MD. Buy it here: amzn.to/2u9TmdE

- *Power vs. Force: The Hidden Determinants of Human Behavior* (Author's Official Revised Edition) by David R. Hawkins, MD, PhD. Buy it here: amzn.to/2uNAu5X

- *The Soulmate Secret: Manifest the Love of Your Life with the Law of Attraction* by Arielle Ford. Buy it here: amzn.to/2u9PQQi

- *The Biology of Belief: Unleashing the Power of Consciousness, Matter & Miracles* (10th-Anniversary Edition) by Bruce H. Lipton, PhD. Buy it here: amzn.to/2v7GlGc

- *Let Magic Happen: Adventures in Healing with a Holistic Radiologist* by Larry Burk, MD, CEHP. Buy it here: http://amzn.to/2hdBdKJ

- *The Blue Zones: 9 Lessons for Living Longer from the People Who've Lived the Longest* (Second Edition) by

Dan Buettner. (The latest edition of this book includes a reading guide designed for groups to discuss and implement many of the simple changes the author advocates for better health.) Buy it here: http://amzn.to/2hdzMvZ

- *Eat Right 4 Your Type: The Individual Blood Type Diet® Solution* by Dr. Peter J. D'Adamo. Buy it here: http://amzn.to/2uNJA2J

- *French Women Don't Get Fat: The Secret of Eating for Pleasure* by Mireille Guiliano. Buy it here: http://amzn.to/2eY3y7d

- Gregg Braden, "Bladder Cancer Dissolves in Less Than 3 Minutes Using the Language of Emotion": youtube.com/watch?v=GUbEgg6GklU

- *Hands of Light: A Guide to Healing Through the Human Energy Field* by Barbara Ann Brennan (Illustrated by Jos. A. Smith). Buy it here: amzn.to/2uKgpPX

- *All Is Well: Heal Your Body with Medicine, Affirmations, and Intuition* by Louise L. Hay and Mona Lisa Schultz, MD, PhD. Buy it here: amzn.to/2u9zR4X

- *The Secret* by Rhonda Byrne (I recommend the unabridged audiobook rather than the book or the movie). Buy it here: amzn.to/2he2mgw

These resources are great, but remember: Don't spend too much time researching and thinking about what you should

## Reflections

do. Life is short and time is of the essence, so start creating new healthy habits without delay!

It is my sincere hope that you can find out what's been going on with you, not only in this life, but also when you were in the womb and even in a past life, from a physical, spiritual, and emotional standpoint. You are not just a bundle of flesh and bone that's living in the here and now; the process of your creation began generations ago. You are the sum of many parts.

If you take away nothing else from this book, please take away this: **do not let traditional medicine, with its potions and poisons, be your only healthcare strategy.** The action I would like you to take is to build your healthcare team to include practitioners *in addition* to your conventional doctors. Most people limit themselves to a lot of well-meaning, well-trained, conventional Western doctors. You don't need any more of them in your life; you probably have enough. Pull together a team of individuals who will heal you using multiple strategies. Build in functional medicine practitioners, health coaches, traditional Chinese-medicine doctors and herbalists, Ayurvedic doctors, and homeopaths. Go find practitioners who have a different philosophy, and surround yourself with people who clearly understand that your spirit is important.

Of course, I would be delighted if you chose me to help you begin, continue, or conclude your journey of self-discovery. It is my principal joy in life to provide companionship to others undertaking their soul journeys, and through the web links this book, you will know how to reach me. Here is a reminder of the gifts I am offering, which together are worth more than $1,000:

1. Free Meditation on Flowers: http://drveronica.com/flowers/

2. Free "Are You Toxic?" assessment: https://drveronica.wufoo.com/forms/are-you-toxic/

3. 50 percent discount on a Health Creation Meditation: https://drveronica.wufoo.com/forms/special-offer-health-creation-meditation/

4. 50 percent discount on a Full Medical Intuitive Reading: https://drveronica.wufoo.com/forms/special-offer-full-medical-intuitive-reading/

5. 50 percent discount on a Single-Question Reading: https://drveronica.wufoo.com/forms/special-offer-single-question-reading/

6. Free "How Healthy Are You?" score: https://drveronica.wufoo.com/forms/how-healthy-are-you/

7. A $50 discount at 23andme.com: www.23andme.com/drveronica

8. 50 percent discount: Living Matrix Health Assessment: https://drveronica.wufoo.com/forms/special-offer-living-matrix-evaluation-297/

## Reflections

However, if you do not choose to work with me, I hope you will find someone else with a medical-intuitive gift, perhaps someone in your own community, who can help you see yourself more clearly.

In case our paths never cross again, I would like to leave you with one final gift: the gift of gratitude and love. I give you my gratitude for having decided to pick up and read this book. I also give you my love because I love what I do, I love people, and the creation of this book has been an act of love from me to you.

CPSIA information can be obtained
at www.ICGtesting.com
Printed in the USA
LVHW052350130523
746859LV00010B/364